MW00604794

Malpractice in Surgery

Patient Safety

Edited by
Oswald Sonntag and Mario Plebani

Volume 6

Michael Imhof

Malpractice in Surgery

Safety Culture and Quality Management
in the Hospital

DE GRUYTER

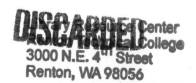

Author

Dr. med. Michael Imhof
Consultant surgeon
Auf der Schanz 96
97076 Würzburg
Germany
Email: praxis@dr-imhof.de

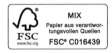

ISBN 978-3-11-027132-4 • e-ISBN 978-3-11-027160-7

Library of Congress Cataloging-in-Publication Data
A CIP catalog record for this book has been applied for at the Library of Congress

Bibliographic information published by the Deutsche Nationalbibliothek
The Deutsche Nationalbibliothek lists this publication in the Deutsche Nationalbibliografie; detailed
bibliographic data are available in the Internet at http://dnb.dnb.de.

Translation: Constantijn Blondel, Leipzig
Typesetting: Compuscript Ltd., Shannon, Ireland
Printing: Hubert & Co. GmbH & Co. KG, Göttingen
Cover image: Comstock/Getty Images

Printed in Germany
♾ Printed on acid-free paper

www.degruyter.com

Contents

Preface

Among humanity's cultural achievements, including science, technology, the arts, religion, and law, medicine plays a central role. Mankind might have accomplished loftier and more aesthetic feats, but among all of them the art of Medicine is the most human, because it does not target beauty, but rather occupies itself with suffering and the inescapability of illness and death, that man is subject to. This way, medicine has accompanied humankind on its development through the millennia. To the extent that man, on his path through history, is continuously confronted with failure, and gets sucked into the abysses of decadence and cultural breakdown, medicine too was accompanied from the very beginning by her mistakes and by her malfunctioning and failure on facing the complexities of disease. Too often, she sinned against her own ethics, due to exorbitant self-overestimation, because of being careless in her dealings with patients and, on occasion, because honorarium became more important than successful treatment. Thus, medicine has always traveled with a close but distrusting companion in the form of law and jurisprudence. Medicine, by necessity, has to live together with its complications, and subsequent charges of failure.

Würzburg, April 2012
Michael Imhof

Abbreviations

ACADEMIA	Antecedents to Cardiac Arrests, Deaths and EMergency Intensive care Admissions
AE	Adverse Event
AGA	American Gastroenterological Association
AHRQ	Agency for Healthcare Research and Quality
AIMS	Australian Incident Monitoring System
AORN	Association of periOperative Registered Nurses
APACHE-II	Acute Physiology and Chronic Health Evaluation II
ASA	American Society of Anesthesiologists
ASRS	Aviation Safety Reporting System
AT III	Antithrombin III
BASIS	British Airways Safety Information System
BDI	Bile Duct Injury
BfArM	Bundesinstitut für Arzeneimittel und Medizinprodukte
BMI	Body Mass Index
BQS	Bundesgeschäftsstelle Qualitätssicherung
CBD	Common Bile Duct
CHD	Common Hepatic Duct
CI	Confidence Interval
CIRS	Critical Incident Reporting System
COPIC	Colorado Physician Insurance Company
CRP	C-reactive Protein
CT	Computer Tomography
DGAI	Deutsche Gesellschaft für Anästhesiologie und Intensivmedizin
DGCH	Deutsche Gesellschaft für Chirurgie
DGGG	Deutsche Gesellschaft für Gynäkologie und Geburthilfe
DGSS	Deutsche Gesellschaft zum Studium des Schmerzes
DMAIC	Define-Measure-Analyze-Improve-Control
EGF	Epidermal Growth Factor
EMG	Electromyography
EOQ	Error Orientation Questionnaire
ERCP	Endoscopic Retrograde Cholangiopancreatography
ESICM	European Society of Intensive Care Medicine
ET	Endoscopic Thyroidectomy

FDA	Food and Drug Administration
FMEA	Failure Mode Effects Analysis
FP	Family Practice
GALT	Gut Associated Lymphatic Tissue
GEMS	Generic Error Modeling System
GMA	German Medical Association
GRM	Generic Reference Model
HMP	Harvard Medical Practice
IATA	International Aviation Transport Association
ICU	Intensive Care Unit
IGF	Insulin-like Growth Factor
IOM	Institute of Medicine
IPOM	Intraperitoneal Onlay Mesh
IQR	Interquartile Range
ISMP	Institute for Safe Medication Practices
ISREC	International Study Group for Rectal Cancer
JCAHO	Joint Commission on the Accreditation of Healthcare Organizations
LA	Laparoscopic Appendectomy
LAD	Lymphadenectomy
LAER	Laparoscopic-assisted Endoscopic Resection
LC	Laparoscopic Cholecystectomy
LDH	Lactate Dehydrogenase
M+M	Morbidity/Mortality
MDK	Medizinischer Dienst der Krankenkassen
MMP	Matrix Metalloproteinase
MODS	Multiple Organ Dysfunction Score
MPSV	Medizinprodukte Sicherheitsplanverordnung
MRCP	Magnetic Resonance Cholangiopancreatography
MRI	Magnetic Resonance Imaging
MRT	Magnetic Resonance Tomography
NASA	National Aeronautics and Space Administration
NBHW	National Board of Health and Welfare
NHS	National Health Service
NHSLA	NHS Litigation Authority
NIH	National Institutes of Health
NPDB	National Practitioner Data Bank
NPSA	National Patient Safety Agency
NRLS	National Reporting and Learning System
NSQIP	National Surgical Quality Improvement Program

OC	Open Cholecystectomy
OMGE	Organisation Mondiale de Gastro-Entérologie
OR	Operating Room
PaSIS	Patienten-Sicherheits-Informations-System
PaSOS	Patienten-Sicherheits-Optimierungs-System
PET	Polyethylene Terephthalate
Peto OR	Peto Odds Ratio
PSA	Prostate-specific Antigen
PSI	Patient Safety Indicators
RCA	Root Cause Analysis
RCT	Randomized Controlled Trial
RF	Radio Frequency
RFID	Radio Frequency Identification
RoD	Relaparotomy on Demand
RSFB	Retained Surgical Foreign Body
SCCM	Society of Critical Care Medicine
SIRS	Systemic Inflammatory Response Syndrome
SIS	Surgical Infection Society
SOFA	Sepsis-related Organ Functional Assessment
TAPP	Transabdominal Pre-peritoneal
TEP	Totally Extraperitoneal
TME	Total Mesorectal Excision
TQM	Total Quality Management
UDAP	Undifferentiated Abdominal Pain
USP	United States Pharmacopeia
WHO	World Health Organization
WSPE	Wrong-side/wrong-site, wrong-procedure, and wrong-patient adverse event

1 Principles of medical malpractice

1.1 Introduction

As can be seen from the rapidly increasing number of complaints about suspected or actual medical errors, the problem of medical malpractice has intensified in the course of the last few decades. In addition, media reports about incorrect treatment with severe consequences for the patient have intensified. Scientific medicine only hesitantly deals with the topic of medical malpractice and patient safety. Yet, the history of medical malpractice reaches far back into antiquity. To deal with this topic, it is necessary to look at the framework within which modern medicine is practiced. By now, the traditionally exaggerated image of the perfect and unerring doctor, curing illness and relieving suffering like a tireless Samaritan, is considered outdated. Modern medicine has become an exceedingly complex service provider, comparable to other high security fields, such as aviation or nuclear technology, and carries its own risks. The scientific and practice-oriented study of mistakes and near-misses is still in its infancy. On a statistical level, the fundamental causes of medical mistakes are being slowly and hesitantly compiled and mandatory guidelines for error management are being implemented within the framework of quality and risk management. There are still barriers to be overcome towards effective prevention of mistakes, which impede an open discussion on malpractice and stand in the way of a preventive culture of constructive criticism.

1.2 Notes concerning the history of medical malpractice

The topic of medical malpractice has accompanied medicine since its infancy. The oldest source of law is found in the so-called Code of Hammurabi, who is said to have lived from 1726 to 1686 BC. This Codex defined professional law for Babylonian physicians and is assumed to derive from Sumerian law texts a thousand years older. This Codex not only defines the honoraria for medical treatment but also codifies drastic repercussions after unsuccessful, or even deficient treatment: for example, it is written about eye operations: "When the physician treats a gentleman, opens an abscess with a knife, and preserves the eye of the patient, he obtains ten shekels of silver. If the patient is a slave, his master will pay two shekels of silver. If the physician opens the eye with a dull knife, kills the patient, or ruins his eye, his hand will be cut off" [1, 2].

Antique medicine reached its breathtaking zenith in ancient Greece, where Hippocrates stood at the birth of an empirical-scientific medical discipline, whose principles are valid even today. Typical examples of scientific medicine in ancient Greece can be found in the so-called "Epidemics": "The physician shall tell what came before, recognize what is, and predict what will be. This art must be practiced. As to diseases, make a habit of two things: to help, or at least to do no harm. The art has three factors, the disease, the patient, the physician. The physician is the servant of the art." [From: http://quotationsbook.com/quote/45518/].

However, already in Greek antiquity, many physicians had a bad reputation. In the Corpus Hippocraticum one author complains that "healing is the most distinguished of the Arts; but due to the ignorance of those who practice it, or of those who frivolously judge it practitioners, it has fallen far behind all the others" [3].

In ancient Rome, for thousands of years, the medical profession, scorned by war-hardened Romans as unworthy of a free man, was only practiced by slaves.

From the 3rd century BC, Greek physicians started settling in Rome. One of them, a surgeon, due to his evident professional failures obtained the moniker "Carnifex" (slaughterer/butcher). Cato the Elder (234-149 BC) particularly despised these Greek physicians: for more than six decades, Rome had managed perfectly well without them. They are a perverted lot, bent on corrupting Rome. Supposedly, they regarded the Romans as barbarians and have nothing in mind, other than to eradicate the Romans with the assistance of medicine. He once wrote to his son: "Never forget that I forbade you to make use of the services of a physician" [4]. Pliny the Elder had little better to say about physicians, their mediocrity, and their greed. In his "Naturalis Historia", he criticized Roman jurisprudence with regard to medical malpractice:

> „Nulla praetera lex, quae puniat inscitiam capitalem, nullum exemplum vindictae. Discunt periculis nostris et experimenta per mortes agunt, medicoque tantum hominem occidisse impunitas summa est".

"There is no law punishing their incompetence (ignorance) if it results in death, and no examples of any penalties imposed. They learn from our precarious situation, and use death to conduct experiments. Only a physician can count on impunity after killing a human being" [5].

Starting around 1200 AD, the fundamentals of Roman law increasingly spread through continental Europe. After the Norman Conquest of 1066, English common law was developed. At the close of the 12th century, during the reign of Richard Coeur de Lion, records were kept in the Court of Common Law and in the Plea Rolls. For example, one early medical malpractice suit in England established that both a servant and his master can sue for damages against a doctor who has treated the servant and made him more ill by employing "unwholesome medicine" [6].

In the late middle Ages, in the year 1532, the German Emperor Charles V issued his "Peinliche Gerichtsordnung" (Constitutio Criminalis Carolina). This court order decreed that, because such questions cannot be decided by a judge, expert witnesses have to be consulted when judging a physician's misdemeanor [7]. With certain provisions, medical malpractice litigation first took off in the USA in 1800 [8].

The American system of medical litigation derives from British Common Law. Common Law refers to laws and legal systems, developed exclusively through legislative statutes or executive decisions of Courts and Judges. Although the principles are similar, state laws governing medical malpractice can vary across different jurisdictions. Thus, medical malpractice law in United States is based on Common law and modified only by legislative actions varying from state to state.

During the last three decades of the 20th Century, the traditional reliance on state courts to draft medical malpractice laws started to change. State legislatures have responded to a number of issues concerning the system of tort claims for malpractice and passed laws changing a number of different aspects of malpractice law, sometimes with dramatic effects. Those statutes are often referred to as "tort reforms" [9]. Some proposals have included the introduction of a contractual model of medical malpractice litigation [10] and put into place a no-fault litigation system similar to worker's compensation, or no-fault automobile insurance [11].

Thus, medical malpractice law in the US has undergone numerous changes in the past three decades. Medical malpractice law and law suits have traditionally been subject to court–mandated common law, but state legislatures have enacted a variety of statutes that change many of those principles. In some states there now exist patient-compensation funds. These funds subsidize payments from traditional malpractice insurance and thereby may reduce insurance premiums.

In Germany, R. Virchow, with his amendments to the penal code of the German Empire, introduced the concept of "malpractice", which he defined as a "violation of the generally accepted rules of medical science". The first medical litigation lawsuit in Germany took place in Berlin, in 1811, and had quite a dramatic case history: Luise Thiele, a 21-year-old woman, was admitted to the Charité hospital in Berlin, because she had, as was said at the time, "succumbed to a frenzy", and refused to eat. She was treated by a Dr. Ernst Horn, who submitted her to the so-called "sack method". This method consisted of putting the patient into a bag, where she had to stay for as long as it took for the raving to stop. The medical record for the case notes that the patient screamed unceasingly, and hence was put into the bag on September 1, 1811. At some time during this day, the patient fell silent. On attempting to release her from the bag, she was found lifeless and resuscitation proved fruitless. Dr. Kohlrausch, the physician in charge of the surgical department and one of Dr. med. Horn's adversaries, lodged a complaint. Thus, on October 26, 1811, the first recorded medical trial was opened before the Berlin Court of Appeal (Kammergericht). At first, because they couldn't lay claim to any medical knowledge, the judges refused to hear the case. The Federal Ministry of Justice, however, insisted on its admittance. The judges, again citing their lack of competence, refused to pass judgment on the value of the sack as a valid medical treatment, and decreed calling expert witnesses - a novelty in Germany at the time. Renowned scientists were entrusted with clarifying whether the sack would reliably exclude an influx of air, and it should thus be considered negligent to confine a human being inside. The witnesses came to the unanimous conclusion that it is not possible to suffocate inside such a sack. Hence, on May 18, 1812, Dr. Horn was finally acquitted [12].

1.3 Defining malpractice

The contemporary definition of malpractice derives from the violation of medical standards: a physician may not perform diagnostic or therapeutic actions that do not comply with established medical standards. He is to consistently act as may be expected from a diligent, conscientious, and experienced physician and he may not violate accepted regulations of medical science [13]. Current jurisprudence equates "diligence exercised" and "standards for medical specialists", defined as the degree of knowledge and competence, validated by practical experience and verified through scientific findings at the time of treatment, that may be demanded from a medical specialist of ordinary competence [14]:

A medical treatment is considered negligent if conventional alternatives, carrying far lower risk and unequivocally promising better results, are available, if a therapeutic procedure is used, that is considered controversial by medical science, or if a diligent physician would no longer be able to take responsibility for application of this treatment. (OLG Köln, VersR 1992, 745).

Medical errors can be roughly categorized as general, individual, and structural-systemic.

Despite numerous definitions of medical error, the topic is currently not yet a topic of generally accepted, interdisciplinary discussion. Rather, definitions of malpractice specific to each discipline and classifications containing characteristics relevant to each specialty are dominating the field, and particular mistakes are generally only examined in the narrow context within which they occur [15]. James Reason [16] characterizes malpractice, or wrongdoing as including all those events, where a planned course of mental or physical action does not have the intended result, to the extent that these failures cannot be attributed to external influences. The integrated perspective on the emergence of mistakes, presented in Reason's root cause analysis, has been widely accepted in research on patient safety. A difference is made between "active failure" and "latent conditions". Active failure is understood to involve mistakes taking place at the human-system boundary, caused directly by humans, the consequences of which are usually directly noticeable.

In medicine, we can differentiate between accidental, involuntary mistakes in an automatic procedure ("slips") and active mistakes, emerging from active conscious thinking ("mistakes"), and latent mistakes [17, 18].

After Rasmussen [19], mistakes occur on three behavioral levels, encompassing skill-based, rule-based and knowledge-based action. These three levels of organization pertain to the degree of conscious control, necessary to perform an action, as well as to the degree of practice and expertise of the actor. Whereas in skill-based actions conscious control is largely deactivated, the subject/the physician/the surgeon needs his full attention to perform knowledge-based actions.

Organizational mistakes, structural deficits, an unsuitable selection of coworkers, or deficiencies in their level of education, can lead to charges of organizational fault. It falls to the art of risk management to eliminate such structural and organizational deficits. Those who supervise their fellow physicians face special requirements, especially with respect to education and advanced training. Only when the standard for medical specialists has been guaranteed on the organizational level, through qualified supervision, a doctor-in-training can be trusted with carrying out certain medical procedures [20]. In addition, the number of specialists within a department must be sufficient to guarantee the continuous supervision of physicians in training. A beginner's operation unsupervised by an experienced physician is a prototypical organizational fault. Together with wrong decisions and administration of incorrect medications, mistakes in handling medical equipment and products are very common. It was determined that in the USA, in 8.4% of all patients treated in a hospital, undesired events took place involving medical products. Despite the high norms and standards for the use of medical equipment, application errors are ubiquitous. Two thirds of the incidents with medical products (infusion pumps, patient monitors, respiratory devices, surgical instruments) are caused by operator error [21].

If a violation of hygienic standards can be proved, this almost always results in the physician or the clinic being held liable, and as a rule alleviates the burden of proof on the patient. In 2008, the German Federal Court of Justice once more tightened the rules governing the physician's liability in case of hygienic deficiencies.

The mere occurrence of a medical incident or of complications, including lethal ones, arising from a surgical procedure, does not automatically justify concluding malpractice. Rather, the patient must prove that a medical error has indeed occurred, and that it caused injury. This explains why patients typically have to fight against lack of evidence. In medicine, causal proof is hard to procure, because the stages of any disease are not subject to linear-deterministic laws of nature. Also, the course taken by disease and recovery cannot be predicted with mathematical-logical certainty. In addition, physicians have to perform their craft on already damaged organisms. Even optimal treatment cannot guarantee success, or even that the condition of the patient will not worsen. In medicine, cause and effect are not linearly related, which is one of the reasons for the asymmetry between the patient as plaintiff, and the physician as defendant. In selected cases, jurisprudence alleviates patients' burden of proof. In some cases, it can be transferred from patient to physician, for example, when a 'gross' medical error can be satisfactorily proved. According to a ruling by the German Supreme Court, this kind of error occurs when a physician unequivocally transgresses tried and tested medical treatment policies, and if the mistake, from an objective medical point of view, taking into consideration prevailing standards of knowledge and education, can no longer be reasonably considered as understandable and responsible on the grounds that, given all this, a physician may not make such an error under any circumstance during treatment (BGH NJW 1983, 2080 (2081)). The burden of proof on the patient may also be alleviated when an examination, which with reasonable certainty would have led to findings such that not reacting to these findings would have meant a gross error, has not been performed. (BGH, VersR 99, 60; BGH, VersR 99, 231; BGH, VersR 99, 1282).

US-American jurisprudence defines medical malpractice as any act or omission committed by a physician during treatment that deviates from accepted norms of practice in the medical community and which causes injury to the patient. The US-American and German/European definitions of malpractice are very similar in their criteria of deviation from accepted norms, and of violating established standards of diligence, and largely coincide.

Medical malpractice is a specific subset of tort law that deals with professional negligence. "Tort" is the Nordic word for "wrong" and tort law is a body of law that creates and provides remedies for civil wrongs as distinct from contractual duties or criminal wrongs [22]. The term "negligence" is generally defined as conduct falling short of a certain standard; the most commonly used standard in tort law is that of a so-called "reasonable person" [23]. The concept of negligence maintains that people should be reasonable and diligent in what they do and, if they are not, will be held responsible for injuries that can reasonably be expected as resulting from their negligence [24]. The most important step in negligence lawsuits in the USA is the injured person's burden of proof in showing that receiving substandard medical care caused their injury. The plaintiff must show that the medical care provided by the physician did not meet the appropriate standards. For example, a specialist must practice medicine at the level of a specialist of ordinary competence in the same field, no matter where in the US they are located.

Medical negligence occurs in a wide variety of forms, including misdiagnosis, failure to make a diagnosis, surgical errors, failure to follow up on a diagnosis with proper treatment, and failure to monitor a patient's vital signs.

"Duty" is a legal concept, which establishes the requirement of a physician, nurse, or other medical professional to treat their patients according to accepted standards of medical care. These standards have been developed over hundreds of years, in order to provide physicians with "guidelines" as to how to treat patients best, given certain symptoms.

1.4 Statistical surveys

The Harvard Medical Practice Study, published in the early 1990s, showed that, each year, 44,000–98,000 Americans die due to medical errors [25, 26]. These numbers form the basis of the pioneering study "To Err is Human: Building a Safer Health System" [27], published by the Institute of Medicine (IOM) a few years later.

Translated into everyday terms, these shocking numbers mean that the number of people dying each day as a consequence of medical errors equals the death toll of a jumbo jet crashing. Although such comparisons are not generally accepted, we still might ask ourselves how much technological, scientific, and financial energy our western societies would expend if in actual fact one jumbo jet crashed on every single day: the media would have a field day and the aviation industry, as well as our governments would spare no effort towards improving aviation safety. However, during the last decades, contemporary medicine has largely suppressed the topic of patient safety. Technical progress and the increasing complexity of modern medicine have created new potential risks: in the past, the risk of a patient falling victim to medical errors or complications was largely determined by the nature and severity of the disease. Due to the wide application of increasingly demanding technology and ever more complex organizational structures, modern medicine now carries its own inherent risks. In the meantime, the topics of medical malpractice and patient safety have become one of the hottest topics within healthcare politics. More recently, in the USA, in direct response to the IOM's 1999 report, the federal Patient Safety and Quality Improvement Act was signed into law on July 9, 2005 [28].

In contrast, Central Europe largely lacks the powerful incentives that reward organizations for displaying due diligence and occupying themselves intensively with medical risk optimization and error elimination. The by now widespread insight that even highly developed expert systems, as well as highly qualified and committed professionals are capable of making mistakes should motivate us to consider any duly recognized risks as a valuable opportunity to learn lessons with regard to increased patient safety. In actuality, grossly negligent individual mistakes are rare. Therefore, in high-risk industries like aviation, or space flight, in maritime environments, and especially in the hospital and the operating theatre, communication and cooperation between the various interacting organizational structures plays a central role. We will come back to these points in later chapters.

According to a European study, we may assume mistakes or adverse events to occur in 8–15% of inpatients each year [29].

According to different international studies, the incidence of adverse events in groups of patients residing in peripheral wards is 10–19% [30, 31]. The Harvard Medical Practice (HMP) study, a population-based survey, estimated that 3.7% of all admissions resulted in an injury prolonging the patient's hospital stay or in a disability at the time of discharge from hospital [25].

Steel et al. asserted a much higher rate of iatrogenic injuries, estimated at 36% of admitted patients [32].

The Robert-Koch-Institute in Germany estimates that ca. 40,000 medical malpractice suits take place each year. In particular, the yearly statistics, compiled by the boards of referees and arbitration committees of the regional medical associations, allow us to make mostly quantitative, but also qualitative statements about the incidence and nature of charges of malpractice. These boards review approximately a quarter of them, roughly totaling 10,000 cases. Since 1979, these statistics are being collected and compiled into a nationwide statistical survey. This anonymized data is collected in the offices of the arbitration committee of the northern German medical association in Hannover. The goal of these surveys is, first and foremost, to establish the incidence of medical errors, in order to be able to draw conclusions about their root causes.

In 2010 for example, 11,016 motions were filed. 7,355 of those resulted in actual decisions confirming or precluding medical malpractice. The total number of charges was 14,079, and 2,232 of those cases, corresponding to 24%, confirmed therapeutical errors or informational deficiency.

The most common complaints were suspected or actual wrongful treatment of fractures, or of arthritis of the major joints, therapeutical errors related to breast cancer, but also regarding laparoscopic intervention, generally in the context of laparoscopic cholecystectomy.

The alliance for patient safety concludes, in their published "Agenda 2007", that 5–10% of hospital patients encounter so-called adverse events. 1% encounters a medical error resulting in injury [33].

Taking into account the 18 million inpatient treatments and operations in Germany, we have to estimate the number of medical errors made in the hospital at ca. 1.8 million.

During the "Conference of head physicians", held in May 2008, the total number of cases involving suspected or actual medical errors, processed by the Medical Service of the Health Funds (MDK), was calculated to be ca. 35,000. In ca. 19,000 cases this led to a medical-juristic clarification, and in 16,218 cases the boards issued a definitive opinion. In other, international, studies, the incidence of adverse events in groups of surgical patients residing in peripheral wards was established at 10–19% [30, 31, 34–38]. Up to 20% of incidents during inpatient treatment involved sudden cardiovascular arrest, myocardial infarction, cerebrovascular accidents, pulmonary embolism, or an unplanned transferal to intensive care due to, for example, sepsis or acute pulmonary or renal failure.

According to the ACADEMIA study, conducted in 68 clinics spread throughout England, Australia, and New Zealand, and involving a mixed group of patients from various medical specialisms, 79% of patients transferred to an intensive care unit following cardiovascular arrest displayed signs of vascular- and pulmonary deficiencies, which had gone undetected in the peripheral ward [39].

According to a current study from the Netherlands, incidents have occurred in 3.8–17% of all inpatient treatments. From 12,121 patients who underwent surgery, 2,033 (16.8%) suffered complications and 6.1% fell victim to mistakes that were subsequently logged in the patients' medical records. 69.5% of these errors had no, or only minor consequences. For 25.2%, further medical intervention was necessary. 4.7% led to permanent damage and 0.6% resulted in patient death [40].

A search through the English language literature in Medline and the Cochrane Library, spanning the years 1965–2011, shows only four original studies occupying themselves with a detailed listing of medical errors and preventable adverse events in primary care. The topic was addressed peripherally in three further studies [41].

Tab. 1.1: Studies describing medical error in primary care [41]

Study	Research purpose	Definition of error	Method	Pertinent results
Primary care studies directly describing medical error				
Bhasale et al. [42]	To describe incidents occurring in general practice	An unintended event, no matter how seemingly trivial or commonplace, that could have harmed or did harm a patient	Self-report by 324 FPs from an Australian watchdog research network, using reply cards.	76% of 805 incidents deemed preventable, in the categories of drug management, non-drug management, diagnosis, and equipment; causes included communication, actions of others, and clinical errors of judgment.
Ely et al. [43]	To describe the causes to which family physicians attribute errors	An act or omission for which the physician felt responsible and which had serious consequences for the patient	30-min interviews with 53 randomly chosen Iowa FPs	53 errors reported: delayed diagnoses, surgical and medical treatment mishaps; causes included physical stressors, the process of care, patient-related factors, and characteristics of the physician.

(Continued)

(*Continued*)

Study	Research purpose	Definition of error	Method	Pertinent results
Dovey et al. [44]	To describe medical errors reported by FPs	Something that should not have happened in one's practice, that was not anticipated, and that makes one say, "I don't want it to happen again"	Self-report by 42 FPs from an American research network, using electronic reports and reply cards.	330 errors reported, 83% involving the health care system and 13% involving knowledge and skills; subcategories were office administration, investigations, treatments, communication, execution of clinical tasks, misdiagnosis, and wrong decisions in treatment.
Fischer et al. [45]	To describe the prevalence of adverse events in a risk management database	Incidents resulting in, or having the potential for, physical, emotional, or financial liability.	Review of incident reports, entered by 8 primary care clinics into a risk management database	Prevalence of adverse events was 3.7 per 100,000 visits, 83% were preventable; categories included diagnostics, treatment, preventive and other errors
Primary care studies peripherally describing medical error				
Holden et al. [46]	To determine patterns of mortality and potential preventive factors		A formal review of all patient deaths in a group of general practices	5.1% of deaths preventable; 2 main categories were the delay of diagnosis and treatment and lack of prevention with aspirin therapy
Gandhi et al. [47]	To evaluate primary care and interactions between specialist physicians.		Surveys taken in an academic medical center	Main issues for doctors were lack of timelines and inadequate content
Britten et al. [48]	To describe the misunderstandings between patients and FPs		Qualitative study analyzing 5 data sources	14 categories of misunderstandings were identified.

In 2008, another systematic review, including eight studies from the USA, Canada, the UK, Australia, and New Zealand, reported a median overall incidence of adverse events of 9.2%, with almost half of them considered preventable.

In this study, data from 74,485 patients was analyzed. The main criteria used in the study were the incidence and percentages of adverse events during inpatient treatment. 43.5% of incidents had no, or only minor consequences. In 7.4% of cases, it led to patient death. Operation–(39.6%) and medication–related (15.1%) events constituted the majority [49]. The median incidence of adverse events was 9.2% (IQR 4.6–12.4%). The median percentage of AEs that was judged preventable was 43.5% (IQR 39.4–49.6%).

The majority of events in this study took place in the operating room (41%) (IQR 39.5–45.8%) or patient wards (24.5%) (IQR 21.6–26.5%). Only 3.1% (IQR 2.7-3.5%) of AEs were located in the complex environment of the intensive care unit. The emergency room accounted for 3.0% (IQR 2.9–3.0) of AEs.

In New Zealand, over 5% of 6,579 patients, admitted to 13 hospitals, were associated with preventable in-hospital events, nearly half of which involved some element of systems failure [50].

Annual reports from Saudi-Arabia, covering the period from 1999–2008, showed a trend in the total number of claims, with 440 cases in 1999 escalating to 1,356 cases by the year 2008. The distribution of guilty verdicts over the different clinical specialisms showed obstetrics taking the lead, with a mean percentage of 25.5% for the duration of the study, followed by general surgery, with a mean percentage of 13.8%. Internal medicine and pediatrics followed the surgical specialisms, with a collective mean percentage of 13.1% and 8.9% [51]. The publication of the Institute of Medicine (IOM) report "To Err Is Human", in the year 2000, caused substantial public concern about medical malpractice. The report estimated that potentially preventable adverse events attributable to medical errors during hospital treatment caused between 44,000 and 98,000 deaths at a total cost of 17 to 29 Billion USD annually.

In 2000, the British Medical Journal dedicated a whole issue to the topic of medical malpractice. In its editorial, it showed that, in the time it takes to read the editorial, eight patients are injured due to an avoidable medical mistake and one of them will die as a result [52].

Outside of the country, little is known of how Japan deals with medical malpractice.

In Japan, with respect to the relationship between physician and patient, a traditional paternalistic paradigm long prevailed. However, since the 1990s, principles of transparency have gained traction, following a scandal with HIV-contaminated blood transfusions [53, 54].

Only a few Japanese law firms specialize in medical litigation. Malpractice cases filed in court, ranging from 200 to 400 nationwide in the 1970s and 1980s, began to increase substantially in the 1990s and in 2004 peaked at 1,110 before a recent decline set in. The overall number of malpractice claims is estimated at 5,000–10,000 claims. Rates of preventable adverse events, as estimated from large-scale reviews of randomly selected medical records in the US and Japan, are roughly comparable [55–57].

Although China has greatly improved its healthcare and medical system, the contradiction between arduous medical tasks and insufficient health resources has so far essentially been unresolved. Considering the complexity and humanitarian nature of medical practice, legislators have put in place a relatively lenient penal system for medical malpractice crimes. Medical-legal research must be encouraged. There are hardly any publications on medical errors, their statistics, and their evaluation. One of them mentions 74 cases of medical error in connection with cancer treatments, in Western China, in the period 2000–2009. The main error sources listed in this study are false diagnoses, ineffective or harmful chemotherapy, and the neglect of complications [58].

From 1/2002 to 9/2008, the Department of Pathology of the Peking University Health Center conducted 275 autopsies in cases where no clear medical cause of death had been established. The majority of cases were a result of natural death. Only in 13.5%, either medical error or negligence was involved [59].

1.5 Summary

In Europe as well as in the USA, the contemporary definition of a medical error encompasses the violation of established standards of both medical conduct and of proper care. In Germany, as well as in the USA, when filing a liability suit, the patient must prove that the physician has made a mistake during treatment and that this has resulted in the patient suffering an injury. The causes of medical errors can be classified as being either individual, or systemic-structural. As a rule, active mistakes are readily identifiable actions leading to visibly adverse results. Latent mistakes must not necessarily have any adverse consequences. In the USA, medical errors in hospitals cause up to 98,000 deaths, and carry a price tag of about 30 billion USD. In Germany, no statistical surveys of the number of medical errors occurring during treatment of inpatients have been completed as of yet. However, cautious estimates show that this number runs up to a total of 1.8 million mistakes and adverse events.

References

[1] The Hammurabi Code and the Sinaitic Legislation. Chilperic, E (ed). London, 1921.
[2] Eckhart, WV. Geschichte der Medizin. Springer, Berlin-Heidelberg-New York, 1998.
[3] Diller, H. Das Gesetz. In: Hippokrates. Ausgewählte Schriften. Philipp Reclam jun., Stuttgart, 1984; p. 120.
[4] Toellner, R. Illustrierte Geschichte der Medizin. Vol. I, Andreas u. Andreas Verlagsbuchhandlung Salzburg, 1986.
[5] Below, KH. Der Arzt im Römischen Recht. In: Münchner Beiträge zur Papyrusforschung und antiken Rechtsgeschichte. München: Beck'sche Verlagsbuchhandlung, 1953.
[6] Hopkins v., Everad. 80 English Reports 1164 (1615). From: Bal, Sonny, B.: An Introduction to the Medical Malpractice in the United States. In: Clin Orthop Relat Res. 2009; 467 (2): 339–347.
[7] Radbruch, G. Die peinliche Gerichtsordnung Kaiser Karl V. von 1532 (Carolina). Stuttgart: Reclam-Universal-Bibliothek, 1967.
[8] De Ville, KA. Medical Malpractice in Nineteenth Century America: Origins and legacy. New York, NY: NYU-Press; 1990.
[9] Budetti, P, Waters, TM. Medical Malpractice law in the United States. In: The Kaiser Family Foundation. 2005; p. 1–5.
[10] Havinghurst, C. Private Reform of tort-law dogma: market opportunities and legal obstacles. Law Contemp. Problems. 1986; 49:143–172.
[11] Johnson, KB, Philips, CA, Orentlicher, D, Hatlie, MJ. A Fault-based administrative alternative for resolving medical malpractice claims. Vanderbilt Law Rev. 1989; 42: 1365–1406.

[12] Carstensen, G. Chirurgie und Recht, In: Häring, R (ed). Chirurgie und Recht, Berlin 1983; p. 3–7.

[13] Neu, J. Ärztliche Sorgfalt, Fahrlässigkeit, Behandlungsfehler, In: Neu, J., Petersen, D., Schellmann, WD (ed). Arzthaftung, Arztfehler, Darmstadt 2001; p. 429–431.

[14] Ulsenheimer, K. Der Behandlungsfehler aus juristischer Sicht: Zivilrechtlicher Schadensersatz - gerichtliche Strafverfahren, In: Wolff, H (ed). Der chirurgische Behandlungsfehler. Teupitzer Gespräche 2001; Heidelberg 2002; p. 3.

[15] Rasmussen, J, Duncan, K, Leplat, J. New Technology and Human Error, Chichester 1986.

[16] Reason, JT. Menschliches Versagen: Psychologische Risikofaktoren und moderne Technologien, Heidelberg 1994.

[17] Reason, JT. Human Error. Cambridge; Cambridge University Press. Using Reason's definition, the IOM (Institute of Medicine) has tried to separate medical errors into two parts: the first part of the definition concerns "error of execution" and the latter part "error of planning".

[18] Kohn, LT, Corrigan, JM, Donaldson, MS (ed). Committee on Quality of Healthcare in America, Institute of Medicine. To Err is Human: Building a safer Health System. Washington DC: National Academy Press; 2000.

[19] Rasmussen, J. Human Errors. A Taxonomy for Describing Human Malfunction in industrial installations, In: Journal of Occupational Accidents, 1982; Vol. 4, No.2–4, p. 311–333.

[20] Schwender, T. Organisationsfehler aus der Sicht des Chefarztes. Gynäkologe 1999; 32:927–932.

[21] Hölscher, U, Laurig, W, Müller-Arnecke, HW. Prinziplösungen zur ergonomischen Gestaltung von Medizingeräten. Bundesanstalt für Arbeitsschutz und Arbeitsmedizin. Berlin, Dresden, 2nd ed. 2008; Internet: www.baua.de).

[22] White, GE. Tort law in America: An Intellectual History. New York, NY: Oxford, V. Press; 2003.

[23] Bal, Sonny, B. An Introduction to the Medical Malpractice in the United States. In: Clin Orthop Relat Res. 2009; 467 (2):339–347.

[24] Budetti, P, Waters, TM. Medical Malpractice law in the United States. In: The Henry J. Kaiser Family Foundation. 2005; http://www.kff.org.

[25] Brennan, TA, Leape, LL, Laird, MM. et al. Incidence of adverse events and negligence in hospitalized patients. Results of the Harvard Medical Practice Study I. N Engl J Med 1991; 324:370–376.

[26] Brennan, TA, Laird, MM. et al. The nature of adverse events and negligence in hospitalized patients. Results of the Harvard Medical Practice Study II. N Engl J Med 1991; 324:377–384.

[27] Kohn, LT, Corrigan, JM, Donaldson, MS. To Err is Human: Building a safer Health system. Washington. National Academy Press, 2000.

[28] Patient Safety and Quality Improvement Act, 119, Stat 424, 2005. In: Kalra, De Gruyter, p. 88.

[29] RAND Cooperation for the European Commissions: Technical report: Improving patient safety in the EU, 2008. URL: www.Rand.Org.com.

[30] Bellomo, R, Goldsmith, D, Uchino, S. Prospective controlled trial of effect of medical emergency team on postoperative morbidity and mortality rates. Crit Care 2004; 32:916–921.

[31] Mangano, DT, Layug, EL, Wallace, A, I. Tateo, I. Effect of atenolol on mortality and cardiovascular morbidity after noncardiac surgery. Multicenter Study of Perioperative Ischemia. Research Group. N Engl J Med 1996; 335:1713–1720.

[32] Steel, K, Gertman, PM, Crescenzi, C. et al. Iatrogenic illness on a general medical service at a university hospital. N Engl J Med 1981; 304:638–642.

[33] Aktionsbündnis Patientensicherheit: Agenda Patientensicherheit 2007, Witten 2007.

[34] Schultz, RJ, Whitfield, GF, LaMura, JJ. et al. The role of physiologic monitoring in patients with fractures of the hip. J Trauma 1985; 25:309–316.

[35] Leidel, BA, Kanz, K.-G. A-B-C-D-E Checkliste verhindert Todesfälle auf Station. In: Notfall Rettungsmed 2010; 13 (8): 775–780.

[36] Smith, GB, Prytherch, DR. et al. A review, a performance evaluation, of single-parameter "track and trigger" Systems. Resuscitation 2008; 79:11–21.

[37] Calzavacca, P, Licari, E, Tee, A. et al. The impact of rapid response system on delayed emergency team activation patient characteristics and outcomes – a follow-up study. Resuscitation 2010; 81:31–35.

[38] Hillman, K, Chen, J, Cretikos, M. et al. Introduction of the medical emergency team (MET) System: a cluster-randomized controlled trial. Lancet 2005; 365:2091–2097.

[39] Kause, J, Smith, G, Prytherch, D. et al. A comparison of antecedents to cardiac arrest, deaths and emergency intensive care admissions in Australia and New Zealand, and the United Kingdom – the ACADEMIA Study. Resuscitation 2004; 62:275–282.

[40] Bosma, E, Veen, EJ, Roukema, JA. Incidence, nature and impact of error in surgery. Br J Surg. 2011; June 27.

[41] Elder, NC, Dovey, SM. Classification of medical errors and preventable adverse events in primary care: A synthesis of the literature. The Journal of Family Practice; November 2002, Vol. 51, No. 11.

[42] Bhasale, AL, Miller, GC, Reid, S, Britt, HC. Analysing potential harm in Australian general practice; an incident-monitoring study. Med J Aust 1998; 169:73–6.

[43] Ely, JW, Levinson, W, Elder, NC, Mainous, AG III, Vinson, DC. Perceived causes of family physicians' errors. J Fam Pract 1995; 40:337–44.

[44] Dovey, SM, Meyers, DS, Phillips, RL, Jr. et al. A preliminary taxonomy of medical errors in family practice. Qual Saf Health Care 2002; 11:233–8.

[45] Fischer, G, Fetters, MD, Munro, AP, Goldman, E.B. Adverse events in primary care identified from a risk-management database. J Fam Pract 1997; 45:40–6.

[46] Holden, J, O'Donnell, S, Brindley, J, Miles, L. Analysis of 1263 deaths in four general practices. Br J Gen Pract 1998; 48:1409–12.

[47] Gandhi, TK, Sittig, DF, Franklin, M, Sussman, AJ, Fairchild, DG, Bates, DW. Communication breakdown in the outpatient referral process. J Gen Intern Med 2000; 15:626–31.

[48] Britten, N, Stevenson, F A, Barry, C A, Barber, N, Bradley, CP. Misunderstandings in prescribing decisions in general practice: qualitative study. BMJ 2000; 320:484–8.

[49] Vries de, EN, Ramrattan, MA, Smorenburg, SM. et al. The incidence and nature of in-hospital adverse events: a systematic review. Qual Safe Health Care. 2008 June, 17 (3):216–223.

[50] Davis, P, Lay-Yee, R, Briant, R. et al. Preventable in-hospital medical injury under the "no fault" system in New Zealand. Qual Safe Health Care. 2003 August; 12 (4):251–256.

[51] Al-Saeed, AH. Medical Liability litigation in Saudi-Arabia. Saudi J Anaesth 2010 Sep–Dec; 4 (3):122–126.

[52] Editorial British Medical Journal BMJ 320; 730; March 2000.

[53] Feldman, E A. HIV and blood in Japan: transforming private conflict into public scandal. In: Feldman, EA, Bayer, R. eds. Blood Feuds: AIDS, Blood, and the Politics of Medical Disaster. New York, NY: Oxford University Press; 1999:59–93.

[54] Feldman, E A. Suing doctors in Japan: structure, culture, and the rise of malpractice litigation. In: McCann, M, Engel, D. eds. Fault Lines: Tort Law as Cultural Practice. Stanford, CA: Stanford University (forthcoming, 2009).

[55] Leflar, RB. The Regulation of Medical Malpractice in Japan. Clin Orthop Relat Res. 2009 February; 467 (2):443–449.

[56] Leflar, RB. Law and patient safety in the United States and Japan. In: Jost, TS (ed). Readings in Comparative Health Law & Bioethics. 2nd ed. Durham, NC. Carolina Academic Press; 2007:124–126.

[57] Sakari, H. Report on the Nationwide Incidence of Medical Accidents: III [in Japanese]. Tokyo, Japan: Japan Ministry of Health, Labour & Welfare; 2006; 18.

[58] Guo, YD, Cai, JF, Chang, YF, Guan, P, Wen, JF. Forensic analysis of 74 tumor related medical malpractice cases. In: Fa Y., Xue Za Zhi. 2010 Jun; 26 (3):192–5.

[59] Xie, ZG, Zheng, J. Autopsy study of 275 medical dispute cases. Zhonghua Bing Li Xue Za Zhi. 2009 Jun; 38 (6):370–5.

2 Errors, incidents and complications in general surgery

2.1 Introduction

The following chapters discuss the complications, risks, and mistakes that may occur during diagnosis and surgical treatment of typical diseases from the field of general surgery. Due to the vast amount of different illnesses and surgical procedures, we must limit ourselves to selected examples taken from the main areas of general surgery. Our discourse will aim at sketching those risks specific to surgery that carry a high possibility of resulting claims of medical malpractice. This special section on general surgery will illustrate the issue of medical malpractice on the basis of examples from everyday clinical practice.

2.2 Medical errors in laparoscopic cholecystectomy

2.2.1 Historical remarks

In 1882, Carl Langenbuch performed the first open cholecystectomy, which was to become the gold standard for the surgical treatment of cholelithiasis during the next hundred years [1]. In 1985, Erich Mühe conducted an endoscopic cholecystectomy using a "surgical tube", as an alternative to the fully invasive procedure [2–4]. The laparoscopic method was popularized by Mouret [5, 6] and Dubois [7], and many countries quickly adopted laparoscopic cholecystectomy (LC) as the procedure of choice. A mere four years after its introduction, laparoscopic cholecystectomy accounted for 90% of all cholecystectomies in the USA [8].

Initially, there was no evidence-based data on LC's effectiveness and safety or about alternative procedures. The problem was not so much the procedure itself, but rather the lack of supporting data: the literature arguing the superiority of LC over open cholecystectomy (OC) did not adequately document LC's safety, effectiveness, or cost savings over alternative therapies. Most of the research published between 1985 and 1999 consists of anecdotal or retrospective case descriptions. As endoscopic surgery gained popularity, OC was no longer performed in adequate number to permit comparison studies. The first attempt to perform the necessary critical review of LC was conducted by the National Institutes of Health (NIH) in a Consensus Conference in 1992 [9]. The transition from open to laparoscopic cholecystectomy has been called the most "precipitous and rapid" of all changes in modern surgical medicine [10].

LC was conceived and popularized not at academic centers but by private clinics [10], and its explosive rate of adoption was driven by market forces [11].

2.2.2 Statistics for medical complications

In the USA, 750,000 cholecystectomies are performed every year [12]. In England, in the year 2005, about 50,000 laparoscopic cholecystectomies were performed within the National Health Service system [13, 14].

In Germany, statistics compiled for the year 2008 by the National Institute for Quality Measurement in Health Care (BQS) show 170,751 cholecystectomies [15], of which 156,288 used a laparoscopic method. In 9,071 cases an intra-operative decision was made to convert to an open procedure. In 969 cases, a bile duct injury occurred, which in 237 instances led to a complete severance of the ductus choledochus, corresponding to about 0.5% of all LC procedures.

Other studies conclude that, with 0.2–0.4%, independently of the surgical method used, the incidence of bile duct injuries remains low [16].

The international literature shows a somewhat different picture of the rate of bile duct injuries following laparoscopic cholecystectomy, with an incidence of 0.5% obtained from aggregate statistics involving 124,433 patients [17].

Numerous other reports have shown that the incidence of bile duct injuries has increased from 0.1%–0.2% during the era of open cholecystectomy to 0.4%–0.7% in the current era of laparoscopic cholecystectomy [18–20].

Reports on the incidence of bile duct injuries (BDI) after open cholecystectomy show numbers in the range from 0.1–0.3% (on average 1 out of 500 cases) [21, 22]. In another publication, the incidence of bile duct injury after laparoscopic cholecystectomy was reportedly between 0.15–0.7% (on average 1 out of 200 cases) [23, 24].

A recent meta-analysis, comparing open and laparoscopic cholecystectomy procedures, once again showed an identical complication rate for both procedures [25].

In the 1990s, England and Germany saw an increase in endoscopic sphincterotomies after LC, which carries a risk of developing pancreatitis [26, 27]. The lack of training and experience with open surgery of the bile ducts may lead to an increased risk of technical errors occurring during complicated bile duct revisions [28]. According to data collected and compiled in the USA by Johns Hopkins Hospital in Baltimore and Indiana University in Indiana, the incidence of injuries to the common bile duct has increased from 0.1–0.2% during the era of open cholecystectomy [17, 29] to 0.4%–0.7% in the current era of laparoscopic cholecystectomy [30–34].

Over the last decade, BDI following LC has become recognized as a major health problem, as evidenced by studies evaluating postoperative management and patients' long-term quality-of-life [19, 35].

Thus, studies currently available do not definitively show if and to what extent the incidence and severity of bile duct injury is increased during laparoscopic cholecystectomy, in comparison with conventional surgery. However, more recent studies, involving 1.6 million cholecystectomies, seem to indicate that, after a learning curve in the 1990s, against expectations, the rate of bile duct injuries following LC has plateaued at

0.5%, and that severe and complex forms of bile duct injury may persist at a higher level well into the future [19, 36, 37].

2.2.3 Complications specific to laparoscopic cholecystectomy

Complications after laparoscopic cholecystectomy can be classified as surgical, general laparoscopic, or cholecystectomy-specific:

Tab. 2.1: Complications following laparoscopic cholecystectomy [14]

General laparoscopic
    Creating the pneumoperitoneum/insertion of the ports
      Intestinal perforation
      Vascular injury – aorta, vena cava, iliac vessels
    Electrosurgical injuries
    Herniation at the port site

Specific to laparoscopic cholecystectomy
    Bile duct injury
      Clipping
      Cut/transection
      Resection
      Electrosurgical
    Hepatic artery injury
    Biliary leaks
    Biliary peritonitis
    Lost gallstones

General surgical complications
    Bleeding
    Infection
    Venous thromboembolism

The pneumoperitoneum has an associated morbidity rate of 0.2% [38]. For 0.2%, complications occur due to insertion of a trocar, or a Veress needle [39, 40]. Most frequently these involve intestinal or vascular injuries, with an incidence independent of the use of either an open procedure or a Veress needle [41, 42]. Hemorrhages at the base of the gall bladder occur with a frequency of ca. 1% [43]. Perforations of the gallbladder are common, occurring in 6–40% of laparoscopic procedures. In up to a third of those cases, no gallstones are retrieved and complications may arise many years postoperatively [44, 45].

Injuries to the biliary tract, often in conjunction with vascular injuries, carry a significantly increased risk of postoperative morbidity and mortality, with lasting impairment of quality of life, often leading to malpractice claims. Their immediate detection and repair are associated with an improved outcome. Litigation after OC is uncommon, and studies available from the USA appear to show a much higher incidence of litigation after LC compared with OC [46, 47].

Tab. 2.2: Biliary tract injuries after open cholecystectomy

Type	Criteria
1	Low CHD stricture with a length of the common hepatic duct stump of >2 cm
2	Proximal CHD stricture – common hepatic duct stump <2 cm
3	Hilar stricture, no residual CHD, but the hepatic ductal confluence is preserved
4	Hilar stricture, with involvement of confluence and loss of communications between right and left hepatic duct
5	Involvement of aberrant right sectorial hepatic duct alone or with concomitant stricture of the CHD

In laparoscopic cholecystectomy, thermic lesions in the extra-hepatic bile ducts, as well as malpositioned clips constitute a special risk. An exact classification, preferably making use of the relevant etiology, the detailed structure of the injury and the therapeutic interval, is a prerequisite for proper surgical treatment of such lesions. For bile duct injuries following an open cholecystectomy, the categorization by Bismuth and Lazorthe in particular is customary [48].

Strasberg et al. comprehensively extended Bismuth's classification by including various other types of laparoscopic extrahepatic bile duct injuries. In order to complement Bismuth's classification, various authors (Bergmann, Neuhaus, Csendes, Stewart et al.) have proposed alternative classification systems that cover the whole spectrum of possible lesions [18].

Tab. 2.3: Classification of iatrogenic bile duct injury

Strasberg's classification (1995) [17]

Type	Criteria
A	Cystic duct leaks or leaks from small ducts in the liver bed
B	Occlusion of part of the biliary tree, almost invariably the aberrant right hepatic ducts
C	Transection without ligation of the aberrant right hepatic ducts
D	Lateral injuries to major bile ducts
E	Subdivided as per Bismuth's classification into E1 to E5

Amsterdam Academic Medical Center's classification (1996) [49]

Type	Criteria
A	Cystic duct leaks or leakage from aberrant or peripheral hepatic radicles
B	Major bile duct leaks with or without concomitant biliary strictures
C	Bile duct strictures without bile leakage
D	Complete transection of the duct with or without excision of some portion of the biliary tree

(Continued)

(*Continued*)

Neuhaus' classification (2000) [50]

Type	Criteria
A	Peripheral bile leak (in communication with the CBD) A1 Cystic duct leak A2 Bile leak from the liver bed
B	Occlusion of the CBD (or right or left hepatic duct, i.e., clip, ligation) B1 Incomplete B2 Complete
C	Lateral injury to the CBD C1 Small lesions (<5mm) C2 Extended lesions (>5mm)
D	Transection of the CBD (or right hepatic duct not in communication with the CBD) D1 Without structural defect D2 With structural defect
E	Stenosis of the CBD E1 CBD with short stenosis (<5mm) E2 CBD with long stenosis (>5 mm) E3 Confluence E4 Right hepatic duct or segmental duct

Csendes' classification (2001) [51]

Type	Criteria
I	A small tear of the hepatic duct or right hepatic branch caused by dissection with the hook or scissors during the dissection of Calot's triangle
II	Lesions of the cysticocholedochal junction due to excessive traction, the use of a Dormia catheter, section of the cystic duct very close or at the junction with the CBD, or to a burning of the cysticocholedochal junction by electrocautery
III	A partial or complete section of the CBD
IV	Resection of more than 10 mm of the CBD

Stewart-Way's classification of laparoscopic bile duct injuries (2004) [52]

Type	Criteria
I	CBD mistaken for cystic duct but recognized Cholangiogram incision in cystic duct extend
II	Bleeding, poor visibility Multiple clips placed on CBD/CHD
III	CBD mistaken for cystic duct, not recognized CBD, CHD, or right or left hepatic ducts transected and/or resected
IV	Right hepatic duct (or right sectorial duct) mistaken for cystic duct. Right hepatic artery mistaken for cystic artery Right hepatic duct (or right sectorial duct) and right hepatic artery transacted

2.2.4 Surgical procedure, and possible causes of errors

During LC, the patient lies on an X-ray table. The surgical team may assume one of two formations: in the American position, surgeons stand to the left of the patient, where-as in the French position, they stand between his/her spread legs. After making an infraumbilical incision, the pneumoperitoneum is created, using mini-laparotomy or a Veress needle. In multiple, studies no statistically significant differences between the use of mini-laparotomy or a Veress needle could be confirmed [53, 54]. In obese patients or in case a preliminary operation has taken place, a supraumbilical route of access may be used. After placing a 10 mm telescopic trocar through the incision in the navel, followed by a diagnostic inspection and introduction of the working trocars under direct vision, the hepatobiliary triangle can be opened up in order to obtain a good overview. At all times, the infundibulum must be used as point of reference, with the surgeon dissecting towards the cystic duct [55]. Correct unclamping of the gallbladder is decisive to assure reliable anatomical identification and to facilitate safe dissection: forceps are used to take hold of the base of the gallbladder in order to lift it so that the hepatobiliary triangle can be tightened. In order to prevent damaging the bile duct, a clear view on the junction between the infundibulum and the cystic duct is essential.

One of the main causes of injury is the misidentification of the common bile duct, the ductus hepaticus communis, or an aberrant bile duct [56]. It has been estimated that over 70% of bile duct injuries can be avoided by correct and conclusive identification of the cystic duct and the cystic artery. There are three critically accepted requirements: first, the hepatobiliary triangle must be clear of fat and fibrous tissue - the common bile duct may not be exposed. Second, the lowest part of the gallbladder must be separated from the cystic plate. The third requirement is to confirm that only two structures enter the gallbladder. Once these three criteria are fulfilled, the critical standard of safety is met, and the cystic duct and artery may be separated [57]. Some authors have described a mechanism for a classic laparoscopic injury in case of a "normal" anatomy of the bil-iary tree, which may occur if there is a superior retraction of the gallbladder. Surgeons may believe that they can see the cystic duct and dissect directly on it, rather than dis-secting on the gallbladder. It is possible to follow down along what is believed to be the cystic duct, whereupon the common bile duct is dissected out, clipped and divided as if it were the cystic duct [58, 59].

Other authors have described a variation on this sequence of events, where faulty anterior and medial traction on the Hartmann's pouch fails to open up the hepatobiliary triangle, thus confusing the cystic duct and the common hepatic duct. The junction of the common hepatic duct is subsequently pulled up into the cystic duct and then clipped and divided.

Any connective tissue bridging the gallbladder's infundibulum and the common bile duct (thereby hiding the cystic duct) is often misinterpreted as tissue covering both of them. Often, the main traction on the infundibulum of the gallbladder is in a cephalic rather than a lateral direction, thus aligning the base of the cystic duct with the com-mon duct and enhancing the illusion that the latter is the cystic duct. Upon initiating the dissection and applying traction to the gallbladder, the common bile duct (adherent to the infundibulum) can become prominent, and the infundibulum can partially or completely hide the cystic duct from view. Thus, the surgeon falls victim to an optical illusion which, to his eyes, clearly shows the - supposed - ductus cysticus, leading him to believe that it merges with the gallbladder. This predisposition towards the kind of misperceptions that underlie these class III injuries is specific to the laparoscopic environment, mainly due to the fact that the surgeon has to work with two-dimensional images. However, the lack of haptic sensory clues also plays a role [56, 60].

Normal variations in the anatomy of the vascular system and the biliary tract constitute additional causes of misinterpretations during surgery.

There are three basic ways the cystic duct may join the biliary system.

Most commonly, the cystic duct merges with the CHD below the junction of the right and left hepatic ducts. Occasionally, the cystic duct enters the right hepatic duct above the junction of the right and left hepatic ducts and below that of the right anterior and posterior hepatic ducts, or enters the right posterior duct where the right anterior hepatic duct joins the left hepatic duct. Rarely does the right posterior duct drain into the cystic duct. The cystic duct is usually short and located away from the center of the hepatic hilum. The cystic artery most often emerges from the right hepatic artery, and occasionally there are two cystic arteries. Injury to the right hepatic artery is a well-recognized complication. Ligation of the right hepatic artery, if accompanied by an injury to the duct, can result in a most complex complication, due to ischemic damage to the right lobe of the liver [61].

It is paramount to a positive prognosis, to diagnose and successfully treat a bile duct injury as quickly as possible, as a rule with use of a combined invasive-endoscopic surgical procedure. Smaller, point-shaped injuries can be splinted or sutured, whereas if the common bile duct is completely severed, surgical intervention is always required. Should transection of the common bile duct be identified during surgery and no loss of substance has occurred, an attempt may be made to create a tension-free end-to-end anastomosis. In case of lesions caused by defects or delayed recognition of the injury, direct suture is, as a rule, no longer possible. In the latter case, localized or even already generalized biliary peritonitis often develops, leading to conditions unfavorable for a bile duct anastomosis. In this case, the preferred treatment is hepaticojejunostomy, using a Roux-en-Y bypass, where the optimum timeframe for reconstruction of the bile duct is debated [62]. The majority of authors recommend primary reconstruction to take place at an early stage [17, 63–67].

Postoperative mortality after hepaticojejunostomy is not insignificant: ascending infections with recurrent cholangitis can cause bilateral cirrhosis and constrictions of the biliary tract. Besides the quality of the reconstructive surgery, we list diffuse peritonitis as the main risk factor for developing late anastomosis-related strictures [68, 69].

2.2.5 Medical malpractice litigation after laparoscopic cholecystectomy

According to their statistics, in the year 2010, review boards heard approximately 32 suits involving suspected or actual medical errors connected with cholelithiasis. The number of malpractice charges processed by specialized lawyers, courts, or medical committees is by far larger. As noted above, according to statistics from the BQS, in Germany, in 2008, 170,751 cholecystectomies were performed, most of the time using laparoscopic methods (156,288). In 9,071 cases, an intraoperative conversion to open

Tab. 2.4: Distribution of injuries occurring during laparoscopic cholecystectomy, as reported in the literature [77]

	No. of cases	Bile duct injury	Vascular injury	Bowel injury	Miscellaneous
Kern (1997) USA	44	61%	9%	9%	14%
Physician Insurers Association of America (1994), USA	324	70%	9%	11%	10%
McLean (2006), USA	104	78%	7%	2%	13%
de Reuver et al. (2008), Netherlands	210	62%	N/A	N/A	N/A
NHSLA, UK (present study)	133	72%	3%	9%	16%

surgery was made. In 969 operations starting laparoscopically, the biliary tract was injured, and in 237 cases the common bile duct was severed. This corresponds to 0.5% and 0.1% of the total number of cholecystectomies respectively. The amount of both judicial and extrajudicial disputes taking place in Germany is not known. According to statistical surveys compiled by review boards, medical error was confirmed in approximately 27 of 100 cases [70]. Anonymized international studies state that 34–49% of surgeons cause injury to the common bile duct at least once in their career [71, 72]. Such injuries often occur after the learning curve has been surmounted, i.e., after having performed 100 cholecystectomies, and therefore can be considered to have been committed by experienced surgeons [73]. The majority of comparative data originates in the USA [74–76]. Although the data encompasses two different decades, legal proceedings are of a surprisingly similar nature.

Litigation after open cholecystectomy is uncommon. In the literature, one report was found that studied such cases. It identified only 49 cases in a 20-year period [78]. De Reuver (De Reuver et al., 2008) looked at BDIs reported to a Dutch insurance company over a period of 13 years. In 80% of case, the injury was diagnosed belatedly. Other authors have reported similar figures, e.g., 86% (McLean, 2006), 83% (Physician Insurance Association of USA), and 80% (Carroll et al.) [79]. The key factor influencing the severity of the outcome is failure to identify the injury once it occurs. A study involving 15 liability insurance funds in the USA, including the Medical Defence Union, together with four from Canada, the UK, and the Republic of Ireland, showed that, in more than two thirds of cases, BDI went undetected during surgery [80]. Delayed recognition of BDI is a frequently used argument for medical malpractice claims.

From 2002 to 2006, the Hamburg institute for forensic medicine analyzed seven cases of death after laparoscopic cholecystectomy [81]. Three cases involved relevant prior medical conditions. In two of those, abdominal adhesions were present. In four cases, complications were proven to have developed as a consequence of LC, with gastrointestinal perforation and BDI occurring twice each.

In one patient, damage to the ductus hepaticus was recognized during surgery. After converting to an open procedure, the BDI was tended to. However, liver abscesses developed post-op, leading to patient death. In another patient, a biliodigestive anastomosis had to be performed four days after LC, resulting from a higher-grade BDI. Prevailing peritonitis necessitated further surgical revisions. Two days after being discharged from hospital, the patient had to be readmitted with symptoms of an acute liver abscess. Subsequently, the patient died from multiple organ failure.

In two other cases, suspected complications during surgery could not be confirmed. One patient died from a fulminant myocardial infarction and one from mesenteric ischemia. There is immense variation of opinion between different reviewers as to how medical errors are assessed both medically and legally, as demonstrated by the following example. Ten completed medical litigation suits were resubmitted to ten highly experienced reviewers. Only one was in full agreement with the original conclusions. Seven cases only showed up to 50% agreement [82]. This phenomenon of similar cases leading to hugely different medical and juridical assessments reflects the relevant experience in Germany. An analysis of decisions on the subject, conducted by the Supreme Court in Germany, shows that, today, contrary to previous jurisprudence, injuries to the common bile duct are considered risks and possible complications inherent in the procedure, rather than a consequence of technical errors [73].

In 2008, for example, one verdict stated that as little as a "subjective sense of certainty" is sufficient reason for a surgeon to forego cholangiography [83]. According to an opinion issued by the Supreme Court, a surgeon must be allowed to base his further course of action on his subjective observation and on his belief of having identified the ductus cysticus [84].

One author, in an editorial in the American Journal of Surgery [85], points out that, with just 0.1–0.5%, the risk of severing the common bile duct is, by all means, acceptable.

As in the USA [86, 87], the theory underlying modern malpractice law in Germany is based on the relationship of trust between the physician and the patient. The patient may expect the physician to provide high quality care, conforming to a well-defined standard. Many examples of human error are regarded as predictable consequences of normal human performance in a high-risk, technology-rich setting, rather than as the result of willful substandard performance. Most high-risk systems, like surgery, have special characteristics "that make accidents [in them] inevitable, even 'normal'. This has to do with the way failures can interact and [with] the way the system is tied together" [88].

Other authors point out that the number and severity of BDIs can be reduced if intraoperative cholangiography is performed [89, 90].

Even though routine intraoperative cholangiography may reduce the incidence of BDIs, it cannot reliably eliminate them [91] and should only be performed if there is any doubt about the patient's anatomy at all. If a BDI occurs, foregoing routine cholangiography does not automatically justify charges of an avoidable error. In addition, with respect to intraoperative cholangiography, the knowledge and experience found in the literature is disputed [55, 92–94].

A study from 2007 [72] could not substantiate any claims to the necessity of intraoperative cholangiography. Surprisingly, it found that cholangiography was able to confirm that misidentification had occurred, but could not prevent the damage done. The study showed that up to 40% of intraoperative cholangiographies are misinterpreted and therefore could not contribute to reliable identification of the structures in the biliary tract. These and similar results have found their way into jurisprudence. In the past, foregoing cholangiography often substantiated malpractice claims, but more recent judgments have not considered it mandatory. In addition, cholangiography carries a risk of damaging structures in the biliary tract. On the other hand, not converting to open surgery is considered an error if, in the presence of unclear or confusing imagery, caused by hemorrhages, adhesions, or anatomical abnormalities, a surgeon does not establish at least "subjective certainty" about the vascular and ductal structures in the hepatobiliary triangle. Before the operation, each patient must be informed about possible conversion to open surgery. Conversion is not considered to be a complication. In addition, as mentioned above, delineating the confluence of the ductus cysticus and the common bile tract, as required by previous standards, is no longer mandatory. Today, the generally accepted standard is the infundibular technique, in which surgeon has to identify the transition between ductus cysticus and infundibulum with sufficient precision [55]. In isolated cases, for example, in the presence of an inflammation or in case of an empyema with risk of gallbladder perforation, the surgeon can deviate from this scheme, without making himself liable to malpractice claims [95]. Fulfilling the three requirements in the critical standard of safety mentioned earlier seems the best way to prevent complications. From a forensic point of view, photo and video documentation must be created when dissecting the vascular and ductal structures in the hepatobiliary triangle [96].

There is a gradual transition from complications inherent in the procedure to culpable medical errors, with space left for differing interpretations by medical review boards, as well as legal points of view. Nevertheless, when the situation is visually confusing or unclear and no serious attempt was made to visually clarify those structures or to convert to open surgery, an accusation of malpractice after structures in the biliary tract are cut is even more likely.

If a laparoscopic procedure is performed by two surgeons, the incidence of bile duct injuries is significantly decreased. Hence, obtaining a second opinion from a colleague may be advisable before any suspicious vital structures are cut [94].

Acute cholecystitis by itself does not indicate conversion to open surgery. The aim should be to perform surgery in an early stage, within 30–72 hours after the onset of symptoms. This approach is associated with both lower morbidity (14–30% vs. 3.4–47.7%) and lower mortality (0 vs. 0–3.5%) rates than interval surgery [97]. The rate of conversion lies between 6–36% and depends on the extent of the inflammation and the specific surgical experience of the surgeon. Here too, experienced medical centers show no difference in the complication rate between laparoscopic and open procedures. In case of acute cholecystitis, foregoing conversion does not substantiate claims of preventable medical error. Only 24–38% of BDIs is recognized intraoperatively and, as a rule, requires immediate conversion. Compared to normal postoperative development, a persisting high bile secretion, fever, shivering, unusually strong pain, elevated levels of transaminase, bilirubin, and the cholestatic parameters, or paralytic ileus, justify suspecting a BDI. Sonography may show the biliary tract to be enlarged and obstructed. Such abnormal findings should be clarified as early as possible, zeroing in on the symptoms with, for example, sonography, CT, MRCP, and ERCP. Failing to conduct such targeted examinations despite presence of these symptoms is generally considered to substantiate claims of culpable medical error. However, a final diagnosis with BDI may often be preceded by a symptom-free period of days or even weeks [98]. If insufficiencies at the stump of the cystic duct are found, laparoscopically fitting a ligature clip or primary wound closure may be successful. Revising any intraoperative lesions in the biliary tract requires an experienced surgeon, especially for defect lesions. In case of doubt, emergency transferal of the patient to a specialized medical center must ensue. The best long-term results have been achieved in specialized hepatobiliary centers [91, 99]. Schmidt et al. [99] report a success rate of only 17% if the BDI is treated by the same surgeon who caused it, against a 94% success rate if the patient is treated by a specialized surgeon.

One of the most frequent complications of surgical treatment of acute cholecystitis is inadvertently opening the gallbladder. Lost gallstones may cause intra-abdominal abscesses. Missing gallstones must be recovered, and the record of the operation must at least document an attempt. If stones cannot be recovered, conversion to an open procedure is not mandatory - foregoing laparotomy does not substantiate claims of malpractice. However, the abdomen must be thoroughly lavaged in order to clear out bile, which can potentially cause an infection, and to flush out at least some of the lost stones [100]. The diagnosis of complications related to lost gallstones is often made after being identified on an X-ray scan. If there is clear documentary evidence and the patient is aware of the perforation, clinicians may be alerted early to the possibility of a gallstone-related complication.

2.2.6 Informed consent

Before cholecystectomy is performed, a preoperative interview must be conducted with the patient, in which information is provided about the nature and severity of the illness, the details, possible risks and complications connected to the operation, but - importantly - also about any alternative procedures and especially about unforeseeable changes to or expansions of the operation. Patients must not necessarily be informed about every conceivable detail, but they must be able to judge the operation's risk, especially as to how it will impact everyday life, quality of life, and, especially, their professional career. This must be communicated to the patient in an intelligible way and, routinely, well in advance of the operation, so that the patient has sufficient time for consideration. In underage patients, permission must be obtained from the patient's legal representative.

2.2.7 Real-life examples

The following examples of decisions made by review boards and courts of law or stemming from individual practice show that malpractice claims are only considered justified if, on finding a confusing or unclear intraoperative picture, no precautions were taken to clarify the anatomical situation or if no appropriate action was taken on noting postoperative symptoms or clinical findings clearly indicating an irregular healing process.

Example 1
58-year-old female patient, with symptomatic cholecystolithiasis. Ultrasound examination shows multiple stones. Ductus hepatocholedochus not enlarged. Highly superficial OR report, describing only the preparation of the ductus cysticus and the a. cystica, without describing its relation to the infundibulum, nor of the threefold clipping of these structures. Histological findings indicate chronic cholecystitis. Postoperative discharge of markedly large amounts of bloody bilious fluid through the drain, in conjunction with high fever and symptomatic cholestasis. ERCP, conducted on the 11th day post-op, showed occlusion of the ductus choledochus by the clips. During revision surgery, all clips are found on the scarred ductus choledochus, in the presence of a 3 cm long defect present. A biliodigestive anastomosis was performed.

Conclusion: Medical error, since the OR report did not show if, and to what extent, preparation of the ductus cysticus or the a. cystica in the vicinity of the infundibulum was performed. No window between artery and ductus cysticus, to further depict structures of the biliary tract if necessary, was created [101].

Example 2
After laparoscopic cholecystectomy, bile fluid with a volume of up to 700 ml a day is discharged through the drain. Further conspicuous symptoms include rapidly increasing levels of liver transaminases and cholestatic parameters. An abdominal CT scan was made only on the 22nd day post-op, confirming large amounts of free fluid inside the abdomen. During the following laparotomy, no extended bile leak was found. No defects in the efferent bile ducts. Post-op, further loss of large amounts of bile fluid through the drain. On the 49th day post-op, ERCP showed truncation of the common bile duct at the site of one of the clips. The following laparotomy verified a large defect in the common bile duct, conforming to Bismuth Type IV, whereupon a biliodigestive anastomosis was performed. Further developments were rife with complications, necessitating six further revision surgeries due to an anastomotic leak, cholangitis, and recurrent scarred stenoses in the area of the anastomosis.

Conclusion: Medical error caused by late diagnosis with a BDI, with poor postoperative outcome, despite imperative early clinical signs and symptoms [102].

Example 3
Laparoscopic cholecystectomy was performed on a 65-year-old female patient with symptomatic cholecystolithiasis. Intraoperatively, poor situational overview and substantial adhesions. An alleged ductus cysticus was identified and obturated. The a. cystica could not be located. Early postoperative symptoms of cholestasis led to another laparoscopy on the 7th day post-op, with the patient having developed sepsis. No sufficient situational overview could be obtained, whereupon the patient was transferred to a university clinic. On arrival, immediate laparotomy was performed, finding a completely resected fork in the bile duct, with exposed stumps of the ductus hepaticus dexter and sinister. The A. hepatica dextra was jammed in the

hepatoduodenal ligament. A biliodigestive anastomosis was performed, followed by longer-lasting postoperative stay in ICU, due to sepsis.

Conclusion: Medical error. The OR report described a large-caliber pulsation in an artery near the gallbladder, incorrectly identified by the surgeon as the a. cystica. The transition from the ductus cysticus to the infundibulum was not dissected. Subjective certainty about the patient's anatomy, suspected by the surgeon himself to be "atypical", was not obtained, resulting in this severe injury to the bile duct.

2.2.8 Summary

By now, laparoscopic cholecystectomy is the gold standard in the surgical treatment of gallstones. The most serious inherent complications are injuries to the biliary tract, although, by now, both the conventional open and the laparoscopic procedure injuries occur at a rate of 0.5–1.0%. In LC, however, there appears a trend towards more serious types of injuries, including defect lesions in the ductus hepatocholedochus. Assessments of medical malpractice in relation to laparoscopic cholecystectomy, by both medical review boards as well as from courts of law, diverge immensely. Routinely securing complete visualization of the ductus hepatocholedochus, from the gallbladder to the ductus choledochus, is no longer mandatory. From a contemporary forensic point of view, intraoperative damage to the ductus hepatocholedochus is treated as a manifestation of the risks inherent in the procedure. The infundibulum technique is the current, generally accepted standard. Liability is particularly likely if postoperative symptoms indicating a lesion in the biliary tract go unrecognized, or if corrective surgery is delayed.

2.3 Risks and possible errors related to minimally invasive or laparoscopic surgery

2.3.1 Introduction

Entry-related risks are a major part of complications arising from laparoscopic procedures that continue to be the subject of medical liability disputes. Many of these complications may have life-threatening consequences, especially if not rapidly recognized and immediately remedied. Continuous documentation of entry-related complications, as well as an exacting analysis of the occurring errors, is required to establish and improve sustainable quality management.

2.3.2 Fundamentals underlying the technical standard and potential errors

In the surgical treatment of a multitude of gastrointestinal diseases, laparoscopic procedures have largely supplanted the open (i.e., conventional) procedures used in the past. As mentioned before, laparoscopic cholecystectomy has become the gold standard for removing gallstones. Experienced surgical centers treat acute appendicitis laparoscopically virtually 100% of the time. A large variety of other diseases of the esophagus, the stomach, the small intestine, and the colon are either treated laparoscopically or at least laparoscopic-assisted, with procedures ranging from, e.g., resections of the esophagus, the stomach, the pancreas, or the colon, up to total colectomy or proctocolectomy for inflammatory diseases of the bowel. Procedures to treat special types of inguinal hernias, other abdominal hernias, and even extensive colectomies for colorectal carcinomas use laparoscopy. Last but not least, minimally invasive laparoscopic techniques have proven beneficial in bariatric surgery.

The main risks of laparoscopic surgery are entry-related complications, which often lead to medical malpractice charges. In the literature, entry-related complications are listed with an incidence between 0.2% and 3.1% [103–108]. Three different laparoscopic entry techniques are available, using either conventional "push-through" type, dilating or so-called "second generation" trocars, each with their own advantages and disadvantages:

1. Closed procedure, the classic technique using a Veress needle and blind insertion of the first trocar.
2. Direct entrance, using a standard trocar, or an optical trocar, without prior creation of the pneumoperitoneum.
3. The so-called Hasson open entry technique [105] involving a minilaparotomy, using a special Hasson trocar.

In a closed procedure, after creating the pneumoperitoneum, certain safety tests must be conducted:

1. Checking motility by moving the Veress needle in all directions.
2. Conduct an aspiration test with a fixed syringe filled with an NaCl solution, followed by:
3. Introduction of a saline solution and renewed aspiration testing. If the needle is fitted correctly, no aspiration of fluid should be possible.
4. In the suction test, on lifting the abdominal wall, fluid is sucked into the abdominal cavity as a consequence of the resulting vacuum.
5. During automatized gas insufflation, both pressure and flow must be constantly monitored. High pressure may indicate a malpositioned needle. Uniform distribution of the gas may be verified visually and by digital palpation or a perfusion scan. The closed technique now proceeds with gentle screwing movements to insert the trocar.

Most surgeons prefer minilaparotomy, followed by open entry. After introducing the optical trocar, the abdominal insufflation pressure is checked visually. This is a very safe method of entry, especially in case of prior operations. A multitude of trocar systems have been developed and are currently available on the market, differing in the material of which they are made (steel/synthetic), valve system and obturator used, and in flexibility. A so-called safety trocar uses a protecting sleeve that slides over the trocar's sharp tip after penetrating into the abdominal cavity. However, even with these safety measures, injuries to the intraabdominal organs cannot be reliably eliminated [109]. Threaded trocars have a sleeve fitted with an external thread and can be introduced into the body without application of axial force. Using a trocar, the incidence of intestinal perforation after blind puncture of the abdominal cavity is between 1:1,000 and 1:2,000. Vessel injuries occur with a frequency between 1:1,300 and 1:2,500 [104, 105, 110–114].

The following important rules for avoiding complications apply:

- When positioning the patient, lordosis must be prevented.
- Locate the entry point away from expected adhesions (e.g., left subcostal).
- Always conduct safety tests after closed entry.
- Convert to open entry after two unsuccessful attempts with the Veress needle.
- Convert to open entry if adhesions are suspected or after prior abdominal operations.
- If necessary, assess mobility of the intestinal loops in the area of the incision with pre- or intraoperative ultrasound examination.
- If an aortic aneurism is suspected, preoperative ultrasound or CT scans must be made.

A study conducted by the US Food and Drug Administration (FDA), involving 629 reports of complications due to use of trocars, reported injury to major vessels in 65%, injury to visceral organs in 29%, and hematomas in the abdominal wall in 5% of cases [115]. 5% resulted in patient death, mostly due to vascular complications. Another study calculated a mortality rate of up to 20% for retroperitoneal vascular injuries [116].

In the upper gastrointestinal tract, typical examples of laparoscopic intervention are cardiomyotomy with semifundoplication to treat achalasia after unsuccessful attempts at dilation, (semi)fundoplication with hiatal grafts in gastric reflux disease, gastropexy, hiatal grafts and semifundoplication for paraesophageal hernias, and laparoscopic gastric resection (wedge resection, submucosal resections, partial gastric resection, and gastrectomies). Especially for benign diseases of the lower gastrointestinal tract, laparoscopic procedures have become a fixed constant. There are no significant differences in morbidity and mortality between open and laparoscopic surgery [117]. Sigmoid diverticulitis is the most frequently operated colonic disease. We must differentiate between fully laparoscopic, laparoscopic-assisted endoscopic resection (LAER), and hybrid conventional-laparoscopic procedures. The literature does not agree on the exact definition of and boundaries between these concepts. Their indications range from inflammatory intestinal diseases, diverticulosis, Crohn's disease, and colitis ulcerosa to resection of colonic adenomas and, in case of functional disorders (dolichocolon, slow transit constipation, rectal prolapse), to resection of colorectal tumors (anterior resection, rectal extirpation). Adherence to oncological standards of practice, as well as maintaining a safe distance to the tumor, is an important indicator [118]. Curative laparoscopic operations are contraindicated for colonic carcinomas if the tumor has spread to different organs, as well as for multiple cancers, emergency surgery, and, possibly, also for very obese patients [119]. In these cases, a conversion rate of about 20% may be expected [119]. A higher chance of survival for the laparoscopic versus the open procedure ("overall survival") has not (yet) been proven [120–122].

Meanwhile, the initial burst of individual case reports claiming port site metastasis on entry during laparoscopic surgery of colorectal carcinomas, with an incidence of 21%, has not been confirmed [123, 124]. These port site metastases were said to be seen, despite the resected tissue having been disposed of [125]. In later series of reports, the rate of port site metastases has clearly decreased. By now, randomized trials show an incidence between 0% and 1.4% [126, 127]. Important measures to prevent port site metastases are optimal insertion of the trocar (only slight peritoneal defects, no slipping out of the needle during the operation), the "no-touch-technique", disposal of resected tissue in an appropriate bag, and diligent cleaning of the trocar with special rinsing solutions.

According to the literature, trocar site hernias occur with a minimum incidence of 0.02% [128] up to a maximum of 7.7% [129]. For example, in 4,385,000 gynaecological laparoscopies, 933 postoperative trocar site hernias were reported [128]. In another study, 0.04% of 1,000 laparoscopic cholecystectomies, that is, in four cases, a trocar site hernia could be verified [130]. About 70% of patients suffering from trocar site hernias develop symptoms or complications, with the rate of incarceration of trocar channel injuries ranging between 13.9% and 16.8% [128, 131]. It is important to prevent trocar site hernias, because, given the small gap, complications involving incarcerations of intestinal segments or the omentum may occur. Since each trocar channel constitutes a potential hernia gap, incarceration of a trocar site hernia may be suspected if postoperative progress should be found suspicious, for instance if ambiguous symptoms, such as vomiting or constipation, develop, possibly indicating ileus. Opinions in the literature differ as to the minimum trocar size for which fascial closure is indicated. Most publications on the topic lack mention of the trocar design. Hence, it is not possible to draw reliable conclusions about the minimum trocar size necessitating fascial closure. Respective recommendations range from 5 mm [132, 133] up to 10 mm puncture size [134–137] and even a recommendation to forego stitches when using expanding dilating trocars [137]. Overlooking mechanical ileus, caused by intestinal incarceration due to a trocar site hernia, substantiates claims of culpable medical error. This is especially the case if no measures were taken to prevent a trocar site hernia from occurring and when, postoperatively, the possibility of, e.g., mechanical ileus was not considered, despite indicative symptoms, and when relaparoscopy or relaparotomy was delayed, that is, after the patient has developed peritonitis or is in advanced sepsis.

The following are some practical recommendations to prevent trocar site hernias:

1. If possible, avoid the median line and the linea alba, on trocar entry.
2. Use the smallest possible trocar diameter.
3. Use dilating trocars.
4. Use visual inspection when closing the abdominal wall and stitching the fascia and peritoneum.
5. When removing the trocar, completely release the CO_2 and open the trocar valve, to prevent segments of the intestine or the omentum from being sucked into the trocar channel.
6. Treat preexisting gaps in the fascia according to standard surgical practice.

If immediately recognized and promptly corrected, intestinal lesions due to trocar placement are generally not considered to be culpable medical complications. Lesions caused by trocars are considered manifestations of the inherent risks in the procedure, as long as the patient was informed preoperatively about the possibility of this complication occurring and when the OR report notes that the appropriate safety tests have been conducted.

Hence, a belated diagnosis substantiates claims of medical error especially if alarming clinical indicators, e.g., high fever, peritonism, paralytic or mechanical ileus, massive leukocytosis, leukocytopenia, elevated inflammation parameters, tachycardia, or tachypnea, were present but no appropriate action was taken.

It is of particular importance to conduct an exact error analysis as well as to continuously document any complications due to trocar entry [107]. Besides vascular and intestinal injuries, thermal injuries prevail after laparoscopic surgery. Often, thermal injuries to the intestines, ureters, or the bladder are not recognized intraoperatively. It frequently takes several days before they cause severe inflammatory complications and perforations [138].

We must also discuss specific complications arising from the use of CO_2 to create the pneumoperitoneum:

If the limits, set at 1L of insufflated CO_2 per minute and 3–4 liters of CO_2 inside the abdomen, and a maximum intraabdominal pressure of 10–15 mmHg, are significantly exceeded, the following complications may occur, some of them life-threatening:

1. Formation of carbon dioxide emphysemas, caused by extraperitoneal insufflation.
2. CO_2 embolisms due to massive intravascular insufflation.
3. Triggering the vasovagal reflex, elevated diaphragm.
4. Pneumothorax due to congenital defects in the diaphragm.
5. Marked increase in CO_2 resorption, with respiratory and metabolic acidosis.

If the intra-abdominal pressure is too high, blood supply to the small and large intestine may be reduced, and cardiac output may be decreased [139, 140]. Ischemic colitis is a rare, but life-threatening complication [141]. A rapid diagnosis is decisive for the prognosis of mesenteric ischemia. Since the clinical symptoms are often nonspecific, the diagnosis is frequently made belatedly.

The most important criteria for diagnosing injuries to major vessels due to laparoscopic entry are:

1. Large amount of blood flowing back through the Veress needle or through the primary trocar.
2. Acute hypotension or asystole.
3. Bleeding in the abdominal cavity.

Patient death has not only been reported after trocar injuries, but also after injuries to the aorta abdominalis caused by the Veress needle [138].

In Germany, as a rule, trocar injuries to the major intraabdominal vessels (aorta, v. cava, v. iliaca) are considered errors, the more so if management of complications was deficient. This is the case if no immediate rigorous vascular surgery was performed to prevent consequential damage (for example, postischemic compartment syndrome) [142].

2.3.3 Real-life examples

Example 1

Laparoscopy-assisted hysterectomy was performed in the gynecology unit of a hospital, on a 53-year-old patient with postmenopausal bleeding. Massive adhesions were found intraoperatively due to multiple prior operations. Their removal caused superficial serosal lesions in an intestinal loop. A surgeon was called in, who sutured the lesions laparoscopically. From the third day post-op, high fever, nausea, vomiting, and hypotension. Due to a meteoric distension of the abdomen, laxative measures had no effect. Since no improvement was seen, a surgical consultative examination was arranged on the fifth day post-op, indicating immediate emergency laparotomy. Intraoperatively, a small perforation of the cecum was found, in conjunction with diffuse peritonitis in all four quadrants of the abdomen. Ileocecal resection was performed, followed by abdominal lavage. The pathological-histological assessment of the dissected tissue showed ischemic necrosis as the cause of the perforation. A diagnosis with diffuse peritonitis at least two, probably three days late. A long (5 weeks) treatment in intensive care was necessary, as well as multiple follow-up resections.

Conclusion: The delayed diagnosis with peritonitis, after the perforation had occurred must be deemed a culpable medical error, rather than the perforation of the cecum. The CO_2-pneumoperitoneum had caused mesenteric ischemia. Due to inadequate documentation, it could not be established whether intraoperative CO_2-pressures had been elevated during insufflation.

Example 2

A laparoscopic-assisted operation to treat acute sigmoid diverticulosis was performed on a 79-year-old patient with arterial hypertonia, atrial fibrillation, dilated cardiomyopathy, diabetes mellitus, and renal failure, who was under long-term treatment with phenprocoumon. During surgery, substantial adhesions were found, caused by multiple prior operations, which were carefully detached. There was a prominently increased tendency to diffuse bleeding. Numerous prior bleedings had been stopped using bipolar coagulation. Sigmoid resection with descendo-rectostomy was performed, using the double stapling technique. Post-op, the patient was monitored on an intensive care station. Immediately after transfer to ICU, the patient's circulation destabilized, despite continuous infusion of high dosages of vasopressors. The abdomen was bulged up. Three times the patient was given red blood cell concentrates. The drain in the Pouch of Douglas required 500 ml of fresh blood. Four hours after admission to ICU, the patient was returned to the operating room for a relaparotomy. The abdomen contained 1.5 liters of fresh blood, spraying from an open artery in the small intestine mesentery, caused by trocar injury. After remedying the bleeding, the abdomen was packed and provisionally closed.

During a second look operation the next day, the bleeding was seen to have stopped, and the abdomen was permanently closed. During further treatment, the patient's circulation remained unstable and he eventually died from his many pre-existing internal diseases.

Conclusion: This case concerned a high-risk patient with limited capacity for physiological compensation due to multiple pre-existing internal diseases. Recognition of the arterial bleeding was delayed. Relaparoscopy took place in a late stadium, when the multimorbid patient was already in an immediately life-threatening state of shock, from which he never recovered.

Example 3

Laparoscopic cholecystectomy was performed on a ca. 60-year-old patient to treat acute cholecystitis. After introducing the Veress needle into the abdomen, the pneumoperitoneum was created. The cholecystectomy was performed using the standard infundibulum technique. On finishing the operation, the trocars were removed under vision. Early post-op, unusually strong and persistent pain developed. Incomprehensibly, the attending physicians did not conduct a clinical abdominal examination. Laboratory tests showed strongly elevated inflammation parameters. An abdominal ultrasound exam was only conducted on the 5th day post-op and showed large amounts of free fluid inside the abdomen. The ensuing laparotomy found diffuse peritonitis, caused by perforation of the small intestine with the Veress needle. After tending to this small injury, the patient was monitored on an intensive care station. In the following period, the existing peritonitis necessitated two more revision laparotomies.

Conclusion: The perforation of the small intestine by the Veress needle is not considered a culpable medical error, but rather its delayed diagnosis and the ensuing peritonitis. In light of the presence of alarming clinical signs, postoperative management was deemed to be deficient.

2.3.4 Summary

Entry-related issues are a major part of the complications and they must be continuously monitored during laparoscopic intervention. Some of them can have fatal, even lethal consequences, and the surgeon must take active measures to prevent that from happening. It is important, not in the least from a forensic point a view, to note and document every single step of the operation, together with the measures taken to prevent entry-related complications. If a complicated intraoperative situation arises, the risk of continuing the laparoscopic procedure must be weighed against the risks associated with laparotomy. After finding an unclear and confusing situs, and if intraabdominal complications are suspected, claims for damages by patients can be prevented only by an early decision to convert.

2.4 Complications and possible errors in inguinal hernia treatment

2.4.1 Introduction

Ca. 10–15% of abdominal surgical interventions are hernia operations. Hence, they are an important cost factor within the health care system. The primary aim of these operations is to reconstruct the dorsal wall of the inguinal canal. A plethora of surgical techniques exists, with competing anterior and posterior procedures, with or without a Lichtenstein repair. It is essential to inform the patient about the various surgical techniques and their advantages and disadvantages prior to the operation. Hernia operations see an increased use of laparoscopy. Despite extensive standardization of the procedure, intra- and postoperative complications leading to liability claims may be expected, with an incidence of ca. 20%.

2.4.2 Fundamentals of inguinal hernia surgery

Inguinal hernia surgery is one of the most frequently performed types of abdominal surgery. In Germany, ca. 230,000 hernia operations are performed each year. In the USA, 86.8% of 696,000 hernia operations documented in 1996 took place on an outpatient basis [143]. Inguinal hernias are classified after Nyhus [144] or after the system devised by the European Hernia Society, which applies to open as well as laparoscopic procedures. Hernias are classified according to location ("L" = lateral", "M" = medial, "F" = femoral, "ML" = combined) and size of the defect (<1.5 cm, 1.5–3 cm, >3 cm) [145].

During the last 25 years, hernia surgery underwent radical changes, especially after the introduction of tension-free surgical techniques, minimally invasive procedures, and also, not unimportantly, due to the increasing importance of economical factors for determining what kind of treatment is indicated. Hernia surgery took off in the 19th century with Bassini's introduction of herniorraphy [146]. Further milestones were Shouldice's method and Lichtenstein's mesh technique [147, 148]. E. E. Shouldice's method, described in 1945, aims at an anatomical reconstruction of the dorsal wall of the inguinal canal by duplicating the thinned fascia transversalis. Additionally, the aponeurotic structures of the m. transversus abdominis and the sinewy parts of the m. obliquus internus are attached to the iliopubic tract or the inguinal ligament [149]. The next step was Stoppa's placing of a preperitoneal mesh [150].

In 1984, researchers at the Lichtenstein Hernia Institute started a project to develop techniques for tension-free repair of hernias. The principle of this method rests on strengthening the inguinal floor with a synthetic mesh, with sufficient overlap between the mesh and the tissue, as well as reconstruction of the inner inguinal ring [151]. The placement of a big prosthesis, made from PET, as described by Stoppa and Warlaumont [152], was further developed, along with the introduction of laparoscopic techniques. Along with developments in laparoscopic surgery, new procedures were suggested, in which the mesh is used as either a plug or a patch.

After creating the pneumoperitoneum and introducing the optical and working trocars, transabdominal pre-peritoneal (TAPP) inguinal hernia repair proceeds by making a crescent-shaped incision in the peritoneum, above the hernia gap, from the plica umbilicalis medialis to lateral of the inner inguinal ring. The peritoneum is dissected, followed by implantation of a non-absorbable mesh. It is important that the mesh covers Hesselbach's triangle completely. Various fixation techniques are in use, e.g., clips or a hernia stapler.

The TEP method is more technically demanding: a periumbilical division in the frontal layer of the rectus sheath is made, followed by blunt dissection of the rear layer of the rectus. A preperitoneal surgical site is created with help of a balloon dissector. The surgical plane is located between the cranially running, epigastric vessels and the caudally located peritoneum. The mesh is placed so that its caudal edge fits closely to the peritoneal fold. In medial hernias, it overlaps the middle line. The gas is released under vision, with the patient located in a foot-down position. With this method, fixating the mesh is not strictly necessary.

2.4.3 Informed consent

Prior to the operation, the patient must be informed about the following risks and possible complications of the procedure:

Tab. 2.5: Risks and possible complications of surgical hernia treatment [153]

General, independent of patient and surgical technique

- Secondary hemorrhage/hematoma
- Infection of the wound
- Vascular injury
- Nerve injury
- Injuries to the spermatic cord and its vessels. Testicular atrophy in men.
- Bladder injuries
- Thromboembolism
- Keloid scars
- Recidivism
- Chronic pain in the groin.

For mesh implants
- Foreign body reactions
- Formation of seromas
- Shrinking of the mesh
- Damage to the sperm ducts due to pressure exerted by the mesh

For laparoscopic techniques
- Hematoma of the abdominal wall, in the vicinity of the trocar port sites.
- Skin emphysema
- Pneumothorax
- Air embolism
- Trocar injuries to the intestines and the blood vessels
- Injury to the peritoneum
- Formation of seromas causing pseudorecidivism

2.4.4 Intra- and postoperative errors and complications

The most frequent injuries when using conventional techniques are to the nerves and to the iliac and femoral vessels, often because they become trapped under the seams on the inguinal ligaments. The following vessels typically are at risk: a. and v. epigastrica inferior, a. and v. iliaca externa, a. and v. femoralis, corona mortis, and a. and v. obturatoria. Injuries to superficial nerves running through the area (n. iliohypogastricus, n. ilioinguinalis, n. cutaneu femoris lateralis) are responsible for postoperative sensory disorders in the respective areas they tend to. Injury to the n. femoralis is rare. If there is clinical proof of injury, the nerve must immediately be revised via microsurgery. If a lesion in the n. femoralis goes unrecognized, intraoperatively or early post-op, and is not immediately corrected on discovery, this substantiates a malpractice claim. If vessels in the spermatic cord structures are injured, an attempt at reconstruction must be initiated in the same operation [154]. The clinical signs of ischemic orchitis typically occur one to three days after a herniotomy and manifest themselves as a painful swelling of the scrotum, often accompanied by fever and leukocytosis. The OR record must show that no damage was done to the spermatic cord structures. If any signs of an insufficient blood supply to the scrotum are noted, a Doppler ultrasound test must be conducted immediately to determine if a revision operation is indicated. Failing to perform revision surgery is considered as a culpable error.

Constriction of the suturing of the inner inguinal ring by the seam created when using the Shouldice technique often leads to insufficient blood supply to the scrotum: the tip of the small finger should just fit through the inner inguinal ring. Mechanical constriction of the inner ring by the seam, compromising the circulation through the groin, substantiates claiming culpable technical error. The vessels in the spermatic cord can also be injured if, during the Lichtenstein operation, they are accidentally caught and get squeezed. In open procedures (Shouldice, Bassini, McVay, Zimmermann), when creating the seam, injuries to the a. femoralis can be avoided by carefully lifting the lower edge of the inguinal ligament, so that a clear view of the femoral vessels below may be obtained. Transversely severing the spermatic cord of a young male with a minor hernia obviously substantiates claims of culpable technical error, because it could have been prevented by exercising due diligence [155].

For very obese patients, in cases of extreme scrotal hernia or during revision surgery, it is increasingly more difficult to identify the ductus deferens. In these conditions, even a meticulously working surgeon can accidentally injure the ductus deferens. In this case, an immediate attempt is made to reconstruct the ductus deferens with a direct suture. This way, permanent access can be achieved in 50–70% of cases [154]. Most bladder injuries occur for sliding hernias and generally, as long as they are recognized and remedied during the operation, heal without further consequences. Intraoperative intestinal injuries do not automatically substantiate claims of culpable medical error. However, liability exists if alarming clinical symptoms, such as fever, leukocytosis, or the development of acute abdomen develop postoperatively, but are not detected, hence delaying the indication for laparoscopy/laparotomy. As described in detail above, the most prominent injuries during laparoscopic surgery are trocar injuries to the intestines, bladder, and blood vessels. The problem of chronic postoperative pain in the groin, which may occur, in various guises, after every possible reconstructive operation, has so far not been solved. Usually, it is caused by nerve irritations due to direct trauma, overstretching, squeezing, bruises, through thermal damage related to coagulation, or a constricting seam, but also due to inflammation processes, triggered and maintained by the material of which the seam is made or by the implanted mesh [156, 157]. The most frequent injuries after an open seam technique are to the n. ilioinguinalis, n. iliohypogastricus and the genital branch of the genitofemoral nerve [158].

It has been postulated that endoscopic hernia repair results in less chronic pain, due to the preperitoneal placement of the mesh [159]. Liem found a lower incidence of pain after endoscopic hernia repair compared with open non-mesh repair. In a randomized trial spanning 5 years, Grant et al. [160] found that, after one year, the incidence of chronic pain was 27%, compared with 36% for the Lichtenstein group. There also was a significant reduction of reported numbness in the groin (18% vs. 40%).

Specialized hernia centers have reported excellent results for endoscopic repair. In a randomized controlled trial, spanning 5 years, Wright could not prove a reduction in pain after an endoscopic procedure (13% vs. 10%). This study showed a higher incidence of testicular pain after endoscopic procedures, whereas groin pain was more common after open repair [161].

A review of randomized controlled trials, comparing endoscopic with open hernia repair using a mesh, showed that the endoscopic approach was associated with reduced persisting pain [162].

In a multicenter study, in which 19 institutes took part, three different laparoscopic techniques (transabdominal preperitonial repair (TAPP), the intraperitoneal onlay mesh (IPOM), and totally extraperitoneal repair (TEP)) were compared in 686 patients with a total of 869 hernias. The average recurrence rate after 15 months was found to be 4.5%. Laparoscopy-related complications occurred for 4.5% of patients. The three methods showed approximately equal effectivity [163].

A Cochrane review showed a 50–70% reduction of the recurrence rate when using a mesh, compared to inguinal hernia repairs without [164].

Another meta-analysis compared hernia repair with and without implantation of a synthetic mesh. It showed significantly less chronic pain by simply reducing the tension between the sutures, when applying the mesh [165].

The incidence of postoperative pain in the groin is, on average, rather high, fluctuating between 18–75% [166–174].

Van Veen et al. [175] studied 300 patients suffering from chronic inguinal pain and compared their long-term development after the Lichtenstein method against the conventional seam operation. They found that three years post-op, only 5–6% of patients still reported pain, this number dwindling to zero after 10 years. In a study involving 2,100 hernia operations in the period from 1995–2009 [176] 318 Shouldice/Bassini operations (15%), 604 Lichtenstein operations (28.4%), 211 TAPP procedures (9.9%), 942 TEP operations (44.3%), and 51 using other techniques (2.4%) were compared. In 6.2% of cases minor complications occurred and 2.4% suffered major complications. Three patients developed bowel obstructions requiring revision surgery, and three meshes needed to be exchanged due to an infection. The total complication rate after seam operations was 8.2%, after the Lichtenstein method 10.8%, after the TAPP method 9.8%, and after TEP 6.0%. In this group, the incidence of complications following TEP was lower than after the Lichtenstein operation (p = 0.001).

At 3.5%, the incidence of major complications after TAPP was found to be significantly higher than after TEP (1.6%). Note that, in both procedures, the majority of complications occurred during the learning curve period, before 1999. In larger studies, the recurrence rate after minimally invasive procedures was found to be below 2% [177]. Other large-scale studies, conducted over a long post-operative period, found recurrence rates of 0.6–7% for the Shouldice technique and 0–0.77% for the Lichtenstein method [178]. Today, a clear trend is seen towards tension-free methods after Lichtenstein, as well as towards the laparoscopic TEP and TAPP procedures. Frequently, however, liability claims arise due to incorrect placement and fixation of the mesh. Opponents of TAPP argue that an operation which is, in principle, extraperitoneal is now transformed into an intraperitoneal operation, which carries typical risks of organ damage and formation of intraabdominal adhesions [179–181]. Prior to the operation, the patient must be informed about the increased risk of injuries to the intraabdominal organs. A technically deficient placement and fixation of the implanted mesh regularly leads to malpractice claims.

For example, one of the most frequent causes of early relapses is insufficient fixation of Cooper's ligament. Many authors describe an increased recurrence rate, one or two years post-op, in terms of early relapses caused by such technical errors. However, their incidence is decreasing as the learning curve is surmounted [182–187]. A too small choice of the mesh (8 x 13cm), hernias through the slit, or misplacement of the clips and tearing of Cooper's ligament are typical examples of avoidable errors [182, 185, 188–190].

Hence, early recurrence of a hernia after endoscopic mesh placement is often caused by a technical error [191]. With TEP, a technically deficient, i.e., insufficient preparation of the preperitoneal space can also cause early relapses. During exsufflation (that is, venting of the gas), the mesh can roll itself up dorsally. A temporary mediodorsal or laterodorsal fixation of the mesh during exsufflation can prevent this. It is most of all important to use a sufficiently large mesh (13 x 15 cm). Moreover, in medial hernias, the mesh must overlap the centerline. Leaving a preperitoneal lipoma can also substantiate claims of culpable error.

It is strongly recommended to avoid tacking or stapling below the iliopubic tract and especially to avoid the triangle of doom and the triangle of pain. To avoid damaging a nerve, it is not recommended to fixate the mesh laterally. If it is intra-operatively detected that a nerve has accidentally been injured, the anchoring device must be removed. Misplaced staplers can also account for nerve irritation and injury.

Postoperative mismanagement - that is, if clinical signs of secondary bleeding, organ and vascular damage, mesh-related complications, or sepsis are present, but are not acted upon with due diligence - accounts for a lot of malpractice claims.

2.4.5 Real-life examples

Example 1

A 60-year-old patient with an ambilateral inguinal hernia underwent TAPP. He was discharged from hospital on the second day post-op. One day later, he was readmitted, with signs of acute abdomen, vomiting, and a fever of more than 39°C. An emergency median laparotomy found mechanical ileus in the small intestine, caused by an incarcerated intestinal loop, permeating the peritoneal incision site from the previous operation, causing an occult perforation in the preperitoneal space. The surface of the small intestine was covered with irremovable plaque. Resection of the small intestine and an end to end anastomosis were performed. The mesh implanted during TAPP was left in situ, and the space between the mesh and the peritoneum was lavaged and drained. Post-op, a persistent septic syndrome, with leukocytopenia and thrombocytopenia, appeared. Three weeks post-op, following a transitory period of clinical improvement, wound dehiscence developed, manifesting as paralytic ileus. The operation uncovered peritonitis in the lower abdomen and an abscess in the recto-uterine pouch. The infected mesh was removed, the site rinsed and drained, and a fleece, saturated with antibiotics, was placed. After this, healing progressed without further complications.

Conclusion: Technically deficient closure of the peritoneum after the initial operation, causing an intestinal loop to be incarcerated between the peritoneum and the mesh, immediately post-op. Given the pre-existing peritonitis, the infected mesh should have been removed during revision surgery on the third day post-op.

Example 2

A 35-year-old male was operated on a right side direct hernia, using the Lichtenstein technique. The very concise OR report noted tension-free closing of the defect and implanting a mesh, sewed in using the Lichtenstein technique. One week post-op, a follow-up visit was necessary, due to intense pain in the operated area. The clinical findings describe pressure pain in the os pubis. There was neither clinical, nor sonographic evidence to suspect recurrence of the hernia. The patient was given an intravenous local anesthetic. Nevertheless, pain persisted with unchanged intensity. During the following period, the patient visited multiple surgeons. One of them conducted a tactile examination of a questionable bulging in the groin. However, an ultrasound examination provided no helpful clues. Ca. one year after the first operation, revision surgery was performed in a specialized hernia center. During the operation, it was found that, in the first procedure, the mesh had been incorrectly fixated and the ramus genitalis of the n. genitofemoralis had been caught by one of the seams.

Conclusion: Incorrect placement and fixation of the mesh during the first operation.

Example 3

A 33-year-old patient was treated for hernia, by placing an extraperitoneal mesh prosthesis. Intense post-op neuralgia occurred near the n. ilioinguinalis and n. genitofemoralis. In a neurosurgical clinic, a microsurgical revision procedure was performed. It became apparent that, during fixation of the mesh with a tacker, the n. genitofemoralis had been caught with one of the staples.

Conclusion: Fixation of the mesh is not necessary in a TEP procedure. Hence, catching the nerve with the seam during fixation of the mesh may be considered a technical error.

Example 4

A 25-year-old patient reported to the outpatient department of a hospital, with twinging pain in the groin. Clinical findings were not documented. After being diagnosed with an inguinal hernia, the patient was informed about the possibility of a TAPP operation. However, diagnostic laparoscopy showed no herniated curvatures in the groin. Nevertheless, a mesh (10 x 15 cm) was implanted at the painful site. A rotary tacker was used to fixate the mesh, and the peritoneal incision was sutured. Postoperative chronic pain in the groin persisted and was unsuccessfully treated with various locally injected painkillers. An MRI scan showed that the mesh had rolled up latero-ventrally. Relaparoscopy showed that it had rolled up in a ball, which was duly removed. During the operation, an inguinal hernia could, again, not be found.

Conclusion: It is questionable whether herniotomy was an appropriate indication for this young man. Since no unambiguous hernia could be felt during initial examination, and because neither a medial nor a lateral hernia was confirmed during laparoscopy, it was concluded that there was no professionally justified indication for such an elaborate procedure.

Example 5

A 21-year-old patient underwent an operation to repair a herniated thigh, using the Lichtenstein technique. When creating the seam in the fascia transversalis, the epigastric vessels were injured. Suturing was attempted, but in doing so, as is written verbatim in the OR report, a vessel running along the lower edge of the inguinal ligament was injured. This violent bleeding was sopped by creating a ligature. Postoperatively, the patient's dorsalis pedis pulse was diligently monitored. As early as the first day post-op, a swelling in the leg was noted, on the side of the operated hernia. Venous duplex sonography found thrombosis in the v. femoralis, continuing to the v. poplitea. The v. femoralis communis in the groin could not be delineated. Subsequent CT angiography found a hematoma in the operated area, with a threadlike flow of contrast fluid near the a. iliaca externa/a. femoralis, as well as extensive thrombosis in the deep veins of the leg. On the second day post-op, the patient was transferred to a specialized center for vascular surgery. He was diagnosed with a severed a. and v. femoralis and immediately underwent surgery. The venous and arterial defects were repaired with a v. saphena magna transplantation, also known as a Dacron graft.

Conclusion: There are no excuses for not detecting the severing of the major transport vessels in the leg during careful final intraoperative examination of the site of the surgery. The patient should have been immediately transferred to the nearest center for vascular surgery. The long-term prognosis of an interrupted arterial and venous circulation in the affected leg improves, the earlier the lesion is detected and treated.

2.4.6 Summary

Inguinal hernia surgery is one of the most frequently performed operations in general surgery. Before the operation, the existence of an inguinal hernia must be assured with a differential diagnosis, so that, e.g., lymphomas, lipomas, thrombosis of the varicose veins of the v. saphena magna, or hydroceles/varicoceles due to diseases of the efferent urinary tract or the female genitalia can be excluded. If an inguinal hernia cannot be unambiguously confirmed, further examinations are necessary, for example, with ultrasound or, if necessary, CT or magnetic resonance tomography. Prior to the operation, patients must be informed in detail about the possible risks and complications associated with the procedure, in particular about the advantages and disadvantages of the various surgical techniques. As before, among the large variety of methods, conventional open procedures and endoscopic-laparoscopic techniques stand opposite each other.

In endoscopic procedures, the most prominent complications are entry-related (trocar injuries) or are caused by the implanted mesh. Treating these injuries generally necessitates conversion to an open procedure. Liability issues may arise as a consequence of technically incorrect placement of the mesh or they may follow from lack of due diligence when observing alarming postoperative symptoms - that is, those symptoms that may indicate irregular postoperative development.

2.5 Complications and errors in the surgical treatment of benign thyroid disorders

2.5.1 Introduction

Thyroid operations are among the most frequent operations in general and abdominal surgery. Thyroid nodules may be expected to develop in 4–7%, in endemic areas even in as much as 35–50% of all adults. Only a small amount of these nodules, ca. 5%, turns out to be malignant. For scintigraphically cold thyroid nodules, a malignancy rate of 15% may be expected. The risk that an asymptomatic nodule is malignant varies between 0.4 and 13% [192]. Surgical procedures for treating thyroid cancers and immunogenic hyperthyreosis (Basedow's disease) are shaped by the radical nature of the diseases. There exist different procedures to treat euthyroid nodular goiter. In the meantime however, there has been an international paradigm change towards more radical resection strategies. Almost without exception, liability cases concern issues related to postoperative hypoparathyroidism or lesions in the n. recurrens.

2.5.2 Fundamentals of the surgical treatment of struma

In the past, the established surgical procedure to treat benign nodular goiter was the method after Enderlen-Hotz [193]. It has now largely been abandoned and superseded by more extensive resections, adapted to the individual case, up to routinely performing a total thyroidectomy. In complete, as well as partial resection operations, mandatory identification of the n. recurrens, considered controversial for the last 100 years, has now been widely replaced by mandatory identification of the relevant nerves, which made its way into the current guidelines.

A substantial amount of analyses, studying the nerves at risk, has verified a decreasing incidence of postoperative paralysis, despite the radical nature of certain procedures [194–199]. Today, many authors endorse total thyroidectomy even in cases of multinodular goiter, because the incidence of postoperative complications after such a radical operation is by all means comparable with that of partial resection [200–202]. For example, after partial thyroid resection due to multinodular goiter, a recent study showed a recurrence rate of 14% during an average follow-up period of 14.5 years [203]. Other authors report recurrence rates between 0% and 14% with postoperative prophylactic treatment with L-Thyroxine and between 10.7% and as much as 43% if no prophylactic medication was given [193–206]. It was furthermore found that secondary surgery, due to recurrence of the struma, is associated with a significantly higher morbidity [196, 207]. It is well-known that insufficient postoperative iodine substitution is not the only cause of a recurrent struma, but can also be traced to, a.o., the production of insulin-like growth factor (IGF-1) and epidermal growth factor (EGF) following an incompletely removed thyroid parenchyma [208–210]. However, complete thyroidectomy, if performed in a specialized clinic, can achieve a complication rate of less than 1%. For example, Delbride et al. [195] report a 0.5% incidence of permanent damage to the n. recurrens and 0.4% hypoparathyroidism in a group of 3,089 thyroidectomies, corresponding to a total complication rate of 0.9%. Zambudio et al. [211] have reported equally low complication rates (0.1%). Hence, due to its low associated morbidity, complete thyroidectomy, performed in specialized medical centers, could be the future standard [199, 212–218].

If recurrent unilateral paresis is present, due to prior surgery, it must be considered if a single unilateral hemithyroidectomy might suffice, and if limited surgery on the contralateral lobe, away from the suspected pathway of the n. recurrens, may be permitted. The standard procedure for treating inflammatory thyroid diseases and Basedow's disease is a near total resection, which leaves just a minimal part of the thyroid of ca. 2 ml. After such an extensive resection, the risk of developing recidivistic hyperthyroidism is far below 5%. Thus, postoperative hypothyroidism, which needs to be treated with substitution therapy, is considered the lesser of two evils [219].

2.5.3 Informed consent

Aside from the general risks inherent in any surgical procedure, the patient must be informed of the possibility of postoperative uni- or bilateral disorders of the vocal cords and thyroid function. The planned surgical procedure, as well as possible alternative methods, must be discussed with the patient.

With regard to complications, not just the risk of recurrence, but especially the consequences specific to uni- or bilaterally recurrent parses, the necessity of post-operative speech therapy, but certainly also the possible consequences for the patient's professional occupation and further life planning must be communicated to the patient, who must also must be informed about a possible tracheotomy or of lifelong replacement therapy with vitamin D and calcium. Before any revision surgery, the enhanced individual risk of recurrent paresis must be discussed.

2.5.4 Remarks concerning the surgical technique

In thyroid surgery, access is most commonly provided through the Kocher incision. At the start of the operation, before parenchymal resection, the n. recurrens is identified. It can be found with relative ease, distal from its intersection with the a. thyreoidea inferior, by medially rotating the thyroid lobes. Most of the parathyroid glands are located in a radius of 1–2 cm around the intersection of n. recurrens and a. thyreoidea inferior. However, results compiled from autopsies have shown that, in 20% of cases, the upper parathyroid glands may be located outside of their typical region, dorsocranial of the intersection of a. thyreoidea inferior and n. recurrens. There is an even larger variation in the location of the lower parathyroid glands: only 40–60% of them lie in the area around the lower thyroid pole, ventrocaudal to the intersection [220]. If circulation through a parathyroid gland appears endangered, it will be cut into smaller parts, and implanted in the m. sternocleidomastoideus.

The issue of identifying n. recurrens and the hyperthyroid glands is not just a surgical-technical question, but most of all a medical-legal question [221–224].

The right n. recurrens is the shorter of the two, due to it being wrapped around the right truncus brachiocephalicus. The left n. recurrens is longer, due to its terminal branch wrapping around the n. laryngeus inferior, below the dorsal aortic arch. At the level of both upper tracheal rings, the nerve passes through the ligament of Berry and, possibly after multiple branching, enters the wall of the larynx, dorsal to the m. cricothyroideus. The n. recurrens can be located both intraligamentary and intrathyroidal. Extralaryngeal branches, usually two or three of them, occur along 60–90% of the nerve's length, dividing above the junction, before terminating in the larynx [194, 225–227].

However, intraoperative neuromonitoring only records the activity of the m. vocalis, which is innervated by the ventral branch of the n. recurrens. Hence, lesions in the dorsal branch cannot be detected via neuromonitoring. More than 20 different locations have been described within the area around the intersection of the a. thyreoidea inferior and the n. recurrens, mainly involving retrovascular, antevascular and inter-vascular pathways [228, 229].

The external branch of the n. laryngeus superior follows a variety of pathways, close to the a.a. thyreoideae superiores. Hence, the upper polar vessels must be dissected close to the capsule. Damage to these nerves often causes specific changes in the voice, for example, loss of the ability to produce high frequencies. If this happens to, e.g., a singer, this may be a career-ending complication.

Because it is not possible, due to its numerous variants, to predict the pathway of the n. recurrens from one specific observation, extensive, vessel-preserving microdissection of the nerve is the current state of the art and is the crucial step of the procedure. Dissection, with preservation of the nerves, necessitates not just an "orienting" visual examination, but almost always involves identification of the structures by extensive surgical-anatomical neural imaging with the help of optical instruments [230, 231]. Preserving, hemostatic techniques, using bipolar coagulation, vessel sealing and - if necessary - ultrasound dissection, must be applied [232]. The anatomical particularities of the locations of the parathyroid glands necessitate targeted identification, which means microdissection of the parathyroid vessels. The long-term consequences of damage to the parathyroid glands - persistent hypoparathyroidism with disrupted calcium and phosphate homeostasis, cataracts, and basal ganglia calcification - are serious disorders, and a satisfactory substitution therapy with vitamin D analogues and calcium is not always possible.

Intraoperative neuromonitoring provides a functional complement to the visual identification of nerves. It electrically stimulates the n. recurrens and simultaneously records a laryngeal electromyogram. If the neuromonitoring signal and EMG are positive, unimpeded postoperative motility of the larynx may be expected with 98% certainty. If the signal is lost, this number is reduced to a 40–80% chance of temporary paresis and 10–30% chance of permanent paresis [233]. Causes of culpable errors include operator errors, unwanted adjustment of the volume control or the stimulating current, as well as malfunctions of the pick-up electrodes. False positives may arise, if the nerve is stimulated proximally to an injured site which causes a normal EMG signal to be recorded. In light of liability issues, it must be kept in mind that neuromonitoring is not a substitute on par with precise extensive dissection of the nerves.

2.5.5 Technical errors and complications

Ca. 60% of complications, such as, for example, recurring paresis and hypoparathyroidism, are typical of the surgical procedure. However, infections (54%), troublesome scars (5%), and unremoved thyroid nodules (4%) are grounds for malpractice claims [223]. Unremoved nodules or persistent postoperative hyperthyroidism in most cases are assessed as a violation of due diligence [223]. If the patient was sufficiently informed prior to the operation, the n. recurrens was properly identified and postoperative management of complications complied with the relevant standards, recurrent paresis is not considered malpractice or lack of due diligence. However, if there are doubts as to whether an intraoperative procedure was indicated, for example, if, when operating a unilateral recurrent goiter, a thyroid lobe that was completely inconspicuous with regard to shape and size was dissected, leading to recurrent paresis, liability issues become prominent. When treating multifocal autonomy, it is also considered a medical error if a thyroid lobe was not sufficiently dissected. In addition, a technical error may be concluded if, when treating a recurrent struma, in the presence of preexisting unilateral recurrent paresis, the n. recurrens was not identified as part of a subtotal resection on the other side.

Postoperative hypoparathyroidism may be considered a culpable medical error if the parathyroid glands were not identified intraoperatively, i.e., when anatomical identification was not even attempted. The OR report must comprehensibly document the location of the parythyroid gland [234] as well as secure preservation of at least two parathyroid glands [235].

In connection with postoperative hypoparathyroidism, it is considered a medical error if an existing susceptibility to tetanus is not taken into account, no laboratory tests of blood calcium levels are conducted, or if the physician in charge of follow-up treatment was not properly informed.

2.5.6 Prospects for new minimally invasive techniques

Endoscopic thyroidectomy with direct cervical entry (anterior or lateral) is considered minimally invasive, whereas endoscopic thyroidectomy with extra-cervical entry (thoracic wall, breast, axillary) is not. Gagner et al. [236] presented the results of 18 endoscopic thyroidectomies, with anterior cervical entry, for solitary nodules. Cougard et al. [237] presented the result of prospectively collected data on 40 patients, which demonstrated the feasibility of the technique. Henry and Sebag [238], Palazzo et al. [239] and Sebag et al. [240] reported on 38 cases where an ET technique with lateral entry was used. Between 2004 and 2007 112 ET's were performed by Slotema et al. [241].

Kitano et al. [242] and Takami [243, 244] and Ikeda [245] presented retrospective cohort studies of axillary entry (63 patients) and entry through the thoracic wall (44 patients). Park et al. [246] performed ET with thoracic entry in 100 patients. As before, ET is primarily indicated for the management of benign thyroid disorders. Many different endoscopic techniques have been described, but so far, due to their substantial technical difficulties and the still undetermined benefits and possible advantages of this techniques, as of yet, none has been universally accepted. These procedures are contraindicated for, e.g., a large struma, if prior cervical surgery took place and in case of previous radiation therapy in the cervical/cervix area. The conversion rate varies between 0% and 13%. Reasons for converting are hemorrhages, difficulties during dissection, size of the lesion, thyroiditis, and tracheal injury. It has yet to be demonstrated that endoscopic thyroidectomy is indeed superior to conventional thyroidectomy.

As far as liability is concerned, the consequences of these new, and in the future possibly standard, surgical techniques can not yet be determined in sufficient detail. It seems probable that entry-related complications will be the most relevant to liability.

2.5.7 Real-life examples

Example 1
Female patient, 71-year-old. Struma operation, with unilateral recurrent paresis, ca. 40 years prior. Current diagnosis: recurrent struma permagna, CT imaging shows it extending from the base of the mouth penetrating deeply into the thorax. Preoperatively existing stridor due to tracheal compression. Intraoperatively the thyroid tissue was seen grown around the stenosed trachea. Also, constriction of the esophagus. The struma reached deeply into a retrosternal direction. Preexisting right-side recurrent paresis. The right thyroid lobe was found to be more enlarged than the left one and was intrathoracically dislocated and subtotally removed, without an attempt to identify the n. recurrens. The contralateral lobe was also removed subtotally, again without identification of the n. recurrens. After removing the endotracheal tube, the patient developed increasing stridor, necessitating reintubation on the evening of the surgery. Due to bilateral recurrent paresis, tracheotomy was necessary, followed by lateral fixation of the vocal cords.

Conclusion: Preoperatively, a plethora of risk factors existed, increasing the risk of postoperative bilateral recurring paresis by orders of magnitude. The operation was performed in a small hospital, which lacked experience in treatment of diagnoses that carry this kind of risk.

The main intraoperative error was that, after dissecting the massively enlarged right side, where a recurring paresis was already present, the contralateral n. recurrens was not identified.

Example 2
After scintigraphic and sonographic imaging, a 38-year-old female patient was diagnosed with struma nodosa, part of it located retrosternally. Whereas size and activity of the right thyroid lobe were found normal, a nodule was seen running in retrosternal direction from the left thyroid lobe. Ultrasound and scintigraphic imaging gave no reason to suspect malignancy. The OR report describes bilateral subtotal resection with extensive preparation of the n. recurrens, under neuromonitoring. No retrosternal part was found. A follow-up scintigraphic examination, once again, showed the larger retrosternal portion of the struma, which had to be removed in a secondary operation.

Conclusion: The operation failed to meet its intended target; one thyroid nodule was incorrectly left in situ.

Example 3

A thyroidectomy was performed on a 60-year-old female patient with multinodular struma and disseminated thyroid autonomy. Imaging had shown a cold nodule to be present. An undetermined, thread-like structure was seen and neuromonitoring was used, under the assumption that it was the n. recurrens. False positive signals were recorded. It was noticed intraoperatively that the neuromonitoring machine was malfunctioning. After exchanging the electrodes, no more signal could be obtained.

During further preparation of the n. recurrens, it was established that it had been ligated and severed along with a branch of the a. thyreoidea inferior. The nerve stumps were microsurgically readapted. Post-op, unilateral recurrent paresis was confirmed.

Conclusion: The malfunctioning of the neuromonitoring equipment was noticed only intraoperatively. The attending physicians should have verified faultless functioning of the equipment. In addition, the n. recurrens was not prepared accurately at the intersection with the a. thyroidea inferior.

2.5.8 Summary

The surgical treatment of benign thyroid disorders has seen a paradigm change. Subtotal resection without identification of the n. recurrens and parathyroid glands - the previous standard procedure - has largely been abandoned and replaced with function- and diagnosis-oriented techniques, as well as more extensive resections and even complete thyroidectomy. The aspects of thyroid and parathyroid surgery most relevant to liability issues are the determination of what procedure is indicated for a benign thyroid disorder, intraoperative identification of the n. recurrens and the parathyroid glands, and postoperative management of complications.

2.6 Complications and errors arising in the diagnostics and treatment of acute appendicitis

2.6.1 Introduction

Clinics and emergency rooms examine numerous people with unspecific abdominal complaints, caused by, or seemingly caused by acute appendicitis - the most frequent cause of acute abdominal pain. Suspected acute appendicitis is the most frequent indication for performing emergency abdominal surgery. The statement that no human should ever again have to die from acute appendicitis, said to have been made by Dieu la Foy in the 19th century, is still a pipe dream. In fact, due to the ambiguity of the symptoms, diagnosis and treatment of acute appendicitis still provides a challenge to the physician. As before, acute appendicitis displays predominantly clinical symptoms and has a large potency for complications, in many cases providing grounds for malpractice claims.

2.6.2 Fundamentals

As early as 1886, Reginald Heber Fitz [247] described the causes, pathophysiology and progress of acute appendicitis, and pleaded for diagnosing and indicating appendectomy as early as possible. Acute appendectomy is the most frequent indication for abdominal surgery, with a lifetime incidence between 7% and 9% [248]. The first open appendectomy, with entry through an incision in the right lower abdomen, was first described in 1894 by McBurney [249]. For the next 100 years, this method would be the standard surgical procedure. The next step in the technical development of appendectomy was to introduce laparoscopy, first done in 1983 by Kurt Semm [250].

The controversies surrounding the preferred surgical procedure for complex appendicitis - laparoscopic or conventional-open - still persist. In contrast to laparoscopic cholecystectomy, which today is the worldwide standard procedure for symptomatic cholecystolithiasis, the standard use of laparoscopic appendectomy is still under scrutiny. Randomized studies have shown a lower rate of local wound infection after laparoscopic appendectomy, but a higher incidence of postoperative intraabdominal abscesses [251]. A Chinese meta-analysis of 44 randomized controlled trials, involving 5,992 patients, found that the incidence of intraoperative bleeding, intraabdominal abscesses, and urinary tract infections was moderately higher after laparoscopic appendectomy, compared to the open procedure. However, these differences were not statistically significant [252]. Memon et al. [253] believed that the carbon dioxide pneumoperitoneum contributes to mechanical diffusion of bacteria inside the peritoneal cavity. However, this claim has not been experimentally verified. Brümmer et al. [254] found a higher risk of intraabdominal abscesses after laparoscopic cholecystectomy than after open appendectomy (0.31% vs. 0.21%).

In 1997, a study, covering all of the USA, compared 7,618 (17.4%) laparoscopic appendectomies with 36,139 (82.6%) open appendectomies (Guller et al.) [255]. For the laparoscopic procedure, shortened postoperative hospital stay (2.06 vs. 2.88 days, $p < 0.001$), lower infection rate (Peto OR 0.5; 95% - CI 0.38–0.66; $p < 0.0001$), lower rate of gastrointestinal complications (Peto OR 0.8; 95% - CI 0.68–0.96; $p = 0.02$), and lower total complication rate (Peto OR 0.84; 95% - CI 0.75–0.94; $p = 0.002$) was found. Another US study, involving 235,473 appendectomies between 2000 and 2005, compared 132,663 open versus 102,810 laparoscopic appendectomies. In this period, the amount of LAs increased from 32.2% to 58.0% ($p < 0.001$) [256].

In contrast, Katkhouda et al. [257] argued that after the learning curve was surmounted, differences between open and laparoscopic appendectomy in the formation of intraabdominal abscesses have disappeared. By now, the mortality rate for acute appendicitis has become smaller than 1% [258]. However, necessity of revision surgery may be expected in ca. 2% to 4% of cases [259]. Identifying the risk factors that impact the likelihood of appendicitis-related complications is a crucial step in treating these patients [260–268].

The National Surgical Quality Improvement Program (NSQIP) studied a group of 4,163 patients, to try to determine correlations between possible postoperative complications and the various preoperative risk factors [269].

Preoperative factors that unambiguously impact mortality included ASA class IV or V, insulin-dependent diabetes mellitus, the patient being classified maximally dependent on a scale rating functional status, a history of chronic obstructive pulmonary disease, pneumonia at the time of surgery, chronic steroid use, bleeding disorders in the medical history, and advancing age.

If a patient complains about right-side lower abdominal pain, the differential diagnosis must make use of standardized abdominal anamnesis and examination forms.

Absence of symptoms (lack of muscular defense, no dysuria) must also be documented. Appendicitis is usually diagnosed on the basis of anamnesis, the clinical signs present, and laboratory values.

In cases of acute appendicitis, when taking the anamnesis, an initially nonspecific lower abdominal pain is usually reported. As the inflammatory irritation to the peritoneum develops, the pain moves beyond the source of the inflammation towards the right lower abdomen within a few hours. Nausea, vomiting and diarrhea may occur, as well as massive meteorism. Measuring the axillo-rectal temperature difference, often encouraged in the past, is no longer considered necessary to making the diagnosis [270]. Specific indicators and pressure points, e.g., McBurney's point, and Blumberg and Rovsing's signs, are tested. A positive psoas sign is a specific indicator for retrocecal appendicitis. As a matter of principle, a complete abdominal examination must include a rectal examination [271]. During abdominal palpation, the location and intensity of any pressure pain may vary and does not necessarily correspond to the severity of the inflammation. Routine laboratory tests often show mild leukocytosis and elevated CRP levels. More severe leukocytosis suggests a ruptured appendix, rather than acute appendicitis.

Often, the clinical picture is ambiguous and unclear. If the anamnesis and the clinical examinations and laboratory tests are not sufficient for a diagnosis, an obligatory ultrasound scan must be made. Unambiguous proof of free abdominal fluid further strengthens the indication for surgery. Presence of a pathological cockade provides a strong argument for surgery. However, the literature shows a sometimes considerable variation in data on the sensitivity of ultrasound sonography [272]. Since technological progress has increasingly facilitated ultrasound imaging of a normal appendix, additional evaluation criteria, e.g., presence of hyperemia in duplex sonography, have been suggested [273].

If, despite carrying out complete diagnostics, it still remains unclear if surgery is indicated, the concept of "active observation" [274] with short intervals between checkups becomes an option. A time schedule for the examinations must be set and documented in the patient's case file. For inpatient treatment, the usual time between examinations is ca. 3 hours. Some clinics use a scoring system in conjunction with active observation [275–277]. For outpatients, this interval is 12 hours [278, 279]. If this type of monitoring is chosen, regular clinical, laboratory, and (if necessary) sonographic examinations must be conducted.

Should these examinations not be carried out, despite persistent or even worsening symptoms, the physician has violated his duty to determine and substantiate a diagnosis, which may lead to a reversal of the burden of proof. It is also a culpable diagnostic error if surgery is performed, despite the presence of preoperative clinical findings speaking against appendicitis, such as acute purulent pyelonephritis, a bladder stone, or hydronephrosis, and no abnormalities of the appendix are found during the operation.

2.6.3 Remarks concerning the surgical technique

As described above, the literature does not contain unambiguous data that determines superiority of laparoscopic appendectomy versus the conventional open technique. The two techniques are not in competition. Today they are, in fact, considered to be of equal value, although laparoscopic appendectomy shows an ever growing tendency towards being established as the standard procedure. "Laparoscopic appendectomy: time to decide", Fingerhut stipulated, as early as 1999 [280]. As before, in highly advanced stages of inflammation, the use of laparoscopy remains to be determined. For one thing, the degree of inflammation is the most important factor in converting to an open procedure and is accompanied by a significantly enhanced mortality during postoperative convalescence. In addition, randomized studies show at least a trend towards higher rates of postoperative abscess formation after laparoscopic appendectomy of a burst appendix [257, 281–283, 284–292]. On these grounds, the most recent Cochrane Review pleads to critically review if laparoscopic appendectomy should be indicated in advanced stages of inflammation [293]. When performing laparoscopic appendectomy, it is important to ensure identification of the cecal pole and to dissect the appendicular artery with the mesoappendix, furnishing it with metal clips or resorbable clips.

When severing the base of the appendix, routine use of a linear surgical stapler is recommended, as the safest method. In advanced inflammatory stages, use of a Roeder's loop may substantiate a medical malpractice claim, since it can slip off or cut through the fragile tissue, which may in turn lead to failure of the appendicular stump [294]. If local or general peritonitis or abscesses are found, a smear must be taken for bacteriological examination, and the abdomen must be lavaged. Whether a burst appendix can be removed laparoscopically is determined exclusively by the experience of the surgeon. A possible abscess in the recto-uterine pouch may not be overlooked. Controversy exists as to what to do if no abnormalities of the appendix are found. In 15–25% of appendectomies, a macroscopically inconspicuous appendix is found [295]. However, despite absence of macroscopic abnormalities, in 60% of cases, neurogenic appendicopathy can be diagnosed on the basis of histopathological results [296]. Hence, it is important in this context that the patient is informed of this possibility, prior to the operation. Searching for a Meckel's diverticulum is mandatory, and the abdominal screening must be documented in the OR report.

2.6.4 Errors and complications

If postoperative abnormalities are noted, the possibility of bleedings in the vicinity of the trocar site or the suture, failure of the Roeder's loop or the surgical staples, but also abscesses near the wound, intraabdominal abscesses, or postoperative ileus should be considered. If postoperative cardiovascular problems like tachycardia or hypotension occur, laboratory tests or sonographic examination must be conducted, so that secondary bleeding may be excluded. A delay in reacting to septic complications, i.e., abscesses like the ones mentioned above, substantiates medical malpractice claims or claims of violation of due diligence.

If, after finding insufficiency of the appendicular stump, accompanied by an intraabdominal abscess, or even diffuse peritonitis, revision surgery is delayed, this can lead to a long and expensive stay in ICU, multiple revision operations and even patient death.

During and after surgery, abnormal findings must be inspected and documented. If reoperation is erroneously delayed, this may lead to a reversal of the burden of proof. In medical liability cases, incorrect preoperative differential diagnoses, belated indication for treatment, as well as errors and deficiencies in postoperative care, take the foreground.

2.6.5 Real-life examples

Example 1

An 18-year-old man was admitted to hospital on the basis of the following clinical anamnesis and laboratory findings: complaints of gastroenteritis, starting five days ago, initially with nausea and vomiting, later with diarrhea. On admission, a bloated abdomen was noted, with strong muscular defense in all four quadrants. Laboratory tests showed a markedly elevated leukocyte count and distinctly elevated CRP levels. The patient had a 38.5°C fever. Due to the meteoric bloating of the abdomen, ultrasound examination provided hardly any insight. The patient underwent surgery 24 hours after being admitted. During the operation, a burst appendix with diffuse peritonitis was found.

Conclusion: The examination on admission had been incomplete, no fine-grained clinical, laboratory, and ultrasound tests had been conducted, and the operation was delayed by one day. These findings count as culpable medical error.

Example 2

A 58-year-old patient with symptoms of acute appendicitis was admitted to hospital and immediately underwent appendectomy. During surgery, a phlegmonous appendix was found retrocecally, which could be dissected only with difficulty. The OR report did not show how the base of the appendix was sutured (stapler or loop). On the third day post-op, the patient was discharged, although CRP levels were still very high at the time. The letter to the patient's general practitioner did not mention required check-up. After leaving the hospital, right side lower abdominal pain persisted. Finally, three months later, the patient was admitted to a different hospital. Ultrasound examination pointed to a local inflammatory process in the right side lower abdomen. A CT scan showed retrocecal fluid retention.

During revision surgery (conventional laparotomy), large amounts of pus were discharged from the abdomen. The cause of the abscess was found to be an insufficient appendicular stump, 4 cm long. There was pathohistological proof of an acute episode of a chronic-recurrent bleeding and a gangrenous inflammation of the burst appendicular stump, in conjunction with a perityphilitic abscess and purulent peritonitis.

At 68%, the chances of an inflamed appendicular stump bursting are particularly high [297]. Potential factors that may promote inflammation of the appendicular stump are due to the limited field of view and lack of three-dimensional vision, but, importantly, also careless dissection of the cecal base with diathermy instruments [298].

Conclusion: In the case described here, poor overview of the surgical site, due to retrocecal adhesion of the appendix, made the operation technically so complex, that an extended appendicular stump was left in situ. In addition, postoperative care had been deficient, since no check-up was indicated, despite very high CRP levels.

2.6.6 Summary

Even today, despite modern imaging, clinical and laboratory diagnostic techniques, 20% of acute appendicitis operations are performed belatedly, that is, when the appendix has already burst. The amount of surgical errors is small, compared with misdiagnoses and errors in determining indications or in postoperative management. Complications specific to laparoscopy can cause severe consequential damage. The physician owes the patient timely recognition and professional postoperative management of such complications.

2.7 Anastomotic insufficiency in the gastrointestinal tract as a frequent source of malpractice claims

2.7.1 Introduction

Within the field of abdominal surgery, anastomotic leaks in the gastrointestinal tract or pancreatobiliary system, with secondary sepsis, is a severe complication and poses an immediate threat to the patient's life. The associated mortality depends on location and size of the leak and can be explained by contamination of the thorax, the mediastinum or the abdomen, with bacteria-infested or tryptic secretions. The therapeutical principle consists of efficient drainage of the fluids, within the context of a therapy appropriate to the diagnosis. Late or ineffectively treated anastomotic leaks often lead to a prolonged and intensive convalescence, with a large potency for complications, and as such are frequently cause for malpractice claims.

2.7.2 Fundamental concepts

In 2001, Bruce et al. [299, 300] published a study called "Systematic review of the definition and measurement of anastomotic leak after gastrointestinal surgery", listing various definitions of leakage of an esophagogastrostomy, as well as of anastomoses in the hepatopancreaticobiliary system and lower gastrointestinal tract.

Due to the multitude of different definitions, the published anastomotic leakage rates vary, e.g., from 3–23% after rectal resection. The reported incidence of fistulas after pancreatic resection varies between 4–40% and between 0–26% after an esophago-gastrostomy [300]. A contrast X-ray exam is not sufficient for early and unambiguous diagnosis with suture failure near the esophagogastrostomy. Cervical anastomotic leaks often give rise to minor clinical symptoms and saliva secretion through the cervical wound.

In contrast, elective small bowel anastomoses show only a small leakage rate. In general, anastomotic leaks are defined as a major defect of the intestinal wall, in the vicinity of a surgical seam, such that there is communication between the intra- and extraluminal compartments. The consensual definition of the International Study Group for Rectal Cancer (ISREC) defines anastomotic leakage as a defect of the intestinal wall at the colorectal or coloanal anastomotic site, leading to a communication between the intra- and extraluminal compartments. The leaks are classified according to their severity, depending on whether active surgical intervention (B) or relaparotomy (C) or minor active surgical intervention (A) is necessary.

The distance between the anastomosis and the anocutaneous line is especially relevant for deep colorectal anastomoses, the critical distance being 5–7 cm [301–303]. In case of an ultra deep anastomosis, located on the pelvic floor, the rate of leakage increases to as much as 30% [304–306]. Similar to physiological wound healing, anastomotic healing occurs in three phases: the inflammatory, exudative phase, the proliferative phase, and the reparative remodeling phase.

These phases overlap to a certain extent. The risk of an anastomotic leak is largest in the inflammatory (day 1–4) and early proliferative phase (day 4–14). Healing is both faster and more reliable in the small intestine than in the colon. This may be because the colon needs a stronger stimulus in order to induce collagen synthesis [307].

Surgical-technical, patient-dependent, or external factors may negatively influence anastomotic healing. Reduced nutritional status and protein deficiency form additional risk factors [308, 309]. Other studies demonstrated a correlation between low albumin levels and anastomotic dehiscence [308, 310]. A study of 44 patients with anastomotic leakage [309] reported a serum albumin level below 35 g/l as a key risk factor. Prolonged surgery, increased blood loss, and the necessity of a transfusion indicate more complicated or difficult operative procedures, which may in turn increase the risk of anastomotic disruption [311–319].

Other studies mention the negative impact of cachexia on the prognosis [320]. Smoking causes vasoconstriction and nitrous oxide hypoxia, which leads to decreased tissue oxygenation and hence negatively influences wound healing. Consequently, less collagen is produced, leading to a demonstrable reduction of the tissue excitability [321, 322]. It was shown that smoking induces an increase in the activity of collagenases, e.g., MMP-1 and MMP-3 [323] Sorensen [324] provided another detailed demonstration of smoking as an independent risk factor for postoperative anastomotic leakage. Besides many other disruptive factors, certain drugs, e.g., immunosuppressive drugs [326], or steroids, negatively influence wound healing, due to their influence on collagen synthesis [325]. Manifest peritonitis also constitutes an independent risk factor for seam failure [327, 328].

Prominent local factors, relevant to surgery, that may promote leakage, are the used suturing technique, formation of an anastomotic hematoma, electrically and thermally induced necrosis, tissue ischemia, contaminations, and, most of all, not performing the anastomosis tension-free [329]. An anastomotic leak may occur early (3–5 days) or later (7–14 days) post-op. Early causes are intraoperative technical problems or mistakes. Late leakage is often caused by systemically relevant factors, such as circulatory disorders, but is especially likely if the anastomosis was performed in a technically deficient and non-tension-free way. A waterproof suture, absence of excessive ischemia in the vicinity of the seam, and presence of as little foreign substances as possible, are prerequisites for an untroubled healing process. Collagen synthesis, which is important for wound healing, primarily depends on sufficient tissue oxygenation [330]. Multi-row sutures, overtly dense spacing between the stitches, and excessively tight knots restrict the blood flow through and oxygenation of tissue near the seam and are accompanied by an increased leakage rate [331]. Performing a tension-free anastomosis prevents longitudinal tension on the seam, and consecutive constriction of the blood flow and therefore is of particular importance. Hence, the two bowel ends must be generously mobilized. Any seam causes inflammation and tissue necrosis. The smaller the inflammatory response and the extent of the necrosis, the quicker the anastomosis will heal and remain free from irritations, improving the quality of the healing process [332]. For this reason, a single row of stitches is used today, when suturing an anastomosis, because an all-coats suture displays better healing behavior [333, 334].

2.7.3 Anastomotic leaks in the upper gastrointestinal tract

A large percentage of people suffering from esophageal cancer also suffer from functional impairments, increasing the risks inherent in surgery. These impairments are partially determined by alcohol or nicotine abuse, as well as cardiovascular disorders. At 15–40%, the 5-year survival rate is, as before, unfavorable [335–341].

Postoperative morbidity (40%) and mortality (10%) rates are very high [342]. Ferri et al. [335] report data, collected from 434 patients, who underwent esophageal resection surgery to treat a squamous cell carcinoma. In this group, technical complications occurred in 22.6%. However, at 3%, anastomotic leakage was rare. Other studies report anastomotic leakage rates between 3.5% and 21% [339–341, 343–346]. The standard procedure is subtotal transthoracic esophagectomy from the right, with creation of a high intrathoracic esophagogastrostomy (the Ivor-Lewis operation) [347]. If the stomach cannot be used for reconstruction, for example, if the patient underwent prior stomach resection, the interposition graft may be taken from the colon, with blood supply from the a. colica sinistra or colica media. Another method uses a supercharged jejunal interposition graft. A cervical esophagogastrostomy carries a higher risk of complications, with leakage rates of 40% and strictures developing in 50% of cases. However, the resulting mortality rate is as low as approximately 5% or less.

Intrathoracic anastomotic leaks with mediastinitis have a high mortality rate of up to 60% [348]. For a long time, surgeons thought that neoadjuvant chemotherapy increases the risk of an anastomotic leak. However, a number of studies were conducted and none of them could confirm this assumption [349–351].

There have been several reports of minimally invasive esophagectomy in high-volume surgical centers [352, 353].

Ben-David et al. [354] report a group of 61 patients who underwent minimally invasive esophagectomy or a hybrid procedure, with prior neoadjuvant chemotherapy. The anastomosis was performed cervically in 81% and intrathoracic in 11% of cases. Three cervical anastomotic leaks developed (5%). None of the intrathoracic anastomoses developed defects.

If an anastomosis is performed, in spite of precarious blood supply to the colonic interposition graft, this constitutes a culpable medical error. However, most culpable errors consist of deficient postoperative management of complications. Signs such as cloudy secretions, leaking from the intrathoracic drain, fever, tachycardia, elevated inflammation parameters, hypotension, or elevation of the renal function parameters, point towards a possible postoperative anastomotic leak. Postoperative atrial fibrillation also may indicate manifestation of an anastomotic leak [355]. In patients with alcohol abuse in their present or past history, postoperative withdrawal symptoms must be distinguished from sepsis-induced changes in the patient's level of consciousness. If an anastomotic leak is suspected, a contrast x-ray exam, with a water-soluble contrast agent, contrast CT/MRT, or endoscopy (carried out by an experienced physician!) must be performed immediately. Intrathoracic anastomotic leaks can in many cases be bridged with stents so that the defect may be adequately and permanently closed. Quite frequently, late discovery of an intrathoracic anastomotic leak leads to malpractice claims, especially if a mediastinal abscess with lethal consequences has developed. For cervical anastomoses, the wound is opened and the secreted saliva drained off.

The number of adenocarcinomas in the esophagocardial passage is steadily increasing. Epidemiological studies show that, in the Western world, the incidence of adenocarcinomas (squamous cell carcinoma) doubles every five to ten years [356]. Siewert et al. [357] established the following classification:

Tab. 2.6: Classification of adenocarcinomas

Type I.	Adenocarcinoma in the distal esophagus, center 1 cm cranial of the gastroesophageal junction.
Type II.	Tumor located within the gastroesophageal junction, 1 cm above to 2 cm below the boundary.
Type III.	Subcardial gastric carcinoma, center more than 2 cm below the gastroesophageal junction.

The prevalence of the associated Barret's esophagus is more than 90% for type one, between 5–10% for type II and less than 1% for type III.

Since type I tumors are esophageal carcinomas, esophagectomy is indicated as a rule. Transthoracic en bloc esophagectomy, with 2-field lymphadenectomy (LAD) and reconstruction with a gastric sleeve (the Ivor-Lewis operation) is the standard procedure.

Type II and type III are true cardiac and gastric carcinomas, where transhiatal extended esophagectomy is the procedure of choice. A Japanese study found this procedure superior to thoracoabdominal resection, with respect to associated morbidity and mortality. The prognosis is the same for both procedures [358]. Lymphadenectomy encompasses the lower mediastinum and a D2 lymphadenectomy. Endoscopic mucosal resection may be indicated for early type I and II carcinomas [359]. For carcinomas of the distal third of the stomach, a subtotal resection suffices [360, 361]. Early carcinomas are increasingly treated by limited resection: the first laparoscopic-assisted Billroth I resection was performed by Kitano [362, 363] in 1999 in order to remove a gastric carcinoma. Until 2003, Kitawaga et al. [364] conducted more than 1,000 laparoscopic-assisted distal stomach resections. Ohgami et al. [365] developed a technique for laparoscopic gastric wedge resection, in which all layers of the gastric wall are removed.

2.7.4 Errors and management of complications

Anastomotic leakage may cause mediastinitis, regardless of the used technique (abdomino-transhiatal or abdominothoracic). Hence, as for esophageal resections, quick action in dealing with complications is mandatory. Smaller leaks can be closed with, e.g., fibrin glue, whereas larger leaks can be taken care of with a fully covered self-expanding metal stent or - since recently - with self-expanding plastic stents. This permanently seals the fistula.

Depending on the underlying disease, postoperative complications may be expected in 20–40% of cases. High-volume medical centers managed to decrease the postoperative mortality rate to less than 3% [366]. After extended gastrectomy, anastomotic leaks develop in up to 15% of cases. This number decreases to well below 10% in high-volume medical centers [367, 368].

If evidence of an early leak is found within the first 24–48 hours post-op, it may be promising to attempt to either seal the leak with stitches or to recreate the anastomosis, because, at this point in time, the tissue has not yet been damaged by inflammation and necrosis, so that it can still provide enough grip to support the seams. Individual concepts must be synthesized from surgical, endoscopic, and invasive strategies in later stadia.

The development of an anastomotic leak as such does not provide grounds for malpractice claims, which, as a rule, usually arise from inadequate and/or suspected or actual belated reactions to alarming clinical symptoms indicating the development of a leak.

2.7.5 Real-life example

Example

A gastrectomy with an intrathoracic esophagojejunostomy was performed on a 58-year-old patient with a Siewert Type III cardiac carcinoma. The OR report stated that the mesentery of the small intestine was shriveled to a high degree, due to scars from prior abdominal surgery. It mentioned that relocating the jejunal limb to the thoracic cavity, to perform a Roux-en-Y anastomosis, was very difficult.

There was no final verification of blood supply to the anastomosis, nor was it examined for leaks. From the third day post-op, high fever and rapid elevation of the inflammation parameters were noted and interpreted as acute abdomen. During relaparotomy, the anastomosis was found to have burst. At the time, diffuse peritonitis and mediastinitis had already developed. Discontinuity resection was performed. The patient developed sepsis and died from multiple organ failure.

Conclusion: Technical error. The main criterion for untroubled anastomotic healing is to create a tension-free seam. Because the intrathoracic anastomosis was performed under tension, this criterion was not fulfilled. A colonic interposition should have been used. In this context, it must be kept in mind that an X-ray examination is only 50% sensitive to detecting or excluding an anastomotic leak [369]. If a leak is suspected, diagnostic endoscopy is a natural candidate, since both the extent of the defect and the degree of blood supply to the tissue can be accurately determined. Diseased wound tissue may be removed and a stent implanted, as necessary, in the same session [370]. It is of most critical importance to monitor and examine any postoperative clinical symptoms. If the healing process is abnormal or problematic, it is, in all cases, mandatory to consider anastomotic leakage. Problems arising from surgery must be reliably excluded in light of other possible differential diagnoses, e.g., pneumonia or infections of the efferent urinary tract. As soon as clinical symptoms, such as fever, persistent pain, paralysis, decreased state of alertness, organ insufficiencies, elevated inflammation parameters, and, not in the least, notable changes in the secretions discharged through the drain (quantity, appearance, smell), appear, immediate steps must be taken to exclude an anastomotic leak. The primary goal of any treatment is to quickly and sufficiently drain the secretions, as well as to prevent the inflammation from spreading further. A secondary target is to maintain and/or reinstate unhampered intestinal passage and assure that nutrition can be again absorbed from the gut as early as possible.

Due the situation sketched above, the mortality rate in case of an inadequately drained leak is significantly higher than 80% [368], which once more stresses the necessity of rapid and rigorous management of complications.

2.7.6 Anastomotic leakage in the lower gastrointestinal tract – errors and risks

After colorectal resection, anastomotic leaks occur with an incidence of 4–26%. Besides systemic and technical factors, the type of resection (left/right hemicolectomy, sigmoid resection, or high/deep anterior resection) is a determining factor. After deep intersphincteric resection of the rectum, with an anastomosis located in the anal sphincter high pressure zone, and without usage of a protective stoma, the leakage rate is upwards from ca. 10% [371]. For deep anastomoses, current scientific consensus dictates placement of a protective stoma on the pectinate line [372].

The principle of a so-called mesorectal excision (TME) consists of resection of the distal mesorectum down to the pelvic floor and represents contemporary concepts of correct oncological treatment. Hida et al. [373] used specimens, cleared of fat, to demonstrate that 20.2% of lesions contained lymph node metastases within 4 cm of the palpable distal margin of the primary tumor. In 1982, Head et al. [374] reported an anastomotic leakage rate of 17.4% after mesorectal excision and suspected that ischemia and disruption of microcirculation in the anastomosis and in the dead space within in the pelvic cavity might play a major role in developing anastomotic leaks. In contrast, Enker et al. [375] reported a leakage rate of only 4% after complete mesorectal excision. Schiedeck et al. [376] reported that after deep anterior resections, secondary surgery was necessary in 1.8% of cases, to take care of an anastomotic leak. When the double-stapling technique is used, the rows should, if possible, meet perpendicular to each other. Additionally, the seam that seals the rectal stump must be placed outside of the circular stapler anastomosis. The risk of a leak developing seems higher for tangential anastomoses. Performing the anastomosis on the frontal side, which is covered with serous membrane and outside of the staples that suture the rectum, is considered the optimal technique. Failing to take proper action if the anastomosis is visibly ischemic is a technical error. When using the double-stapling technique, any contact between the row of staples and bipolar currents must be strictly prevented, since this may lead to an uncontrolled current flow into the tissue, with extreme heat generation and thermal necrosis of the tissue and ensuing anastomotic leakage. In addition, strict care must be taken to prevent fat (appendices epiploica) from getting caught in the seam. After ejecting the cartridge, it must be checked if both mucosal rings are intact. This must be documented in the OR report. During the operation, it is routinely checked if the anastomosis is sealed, so that leaks at the site of the staples may be recognized and corrected in a sufficiently early stage. Placing a drain near the anastomosis cannot prevent an anastomotic leak, but a correctly placed drain can sometimes keep a leak under control without the need of corrective surgery. Laparoscopic colon resection techniques are on the rise.

Laparoscopic colon surgery was first reported in 1991 [377]. Current evidence suggests that, for rectal cancer, laparoscopic resection is beneficial to the patient, due to earlier return of bowel function, reduced blood loss, and shorter stay in the hospital. The oncological prognosis is comparable to open surgery. However, the evidence relies mainly on case studies and comparative reviews, with only a few RCTs. The findings agree with the Cochrane review from 2006 on short-term outcome of laparoscopic versus open TME for rectal cancer [378].

As in the gastrointestinal tract, fever, paralytic ileus, progressive reduction of cardiac and renal function, and especially elevated inflammation parameters are warning signs for an anastomotic leak. Prolonged postoperative paralytic ileus is often interpreted as a physiological reaction. The actual cause – the anastomotic leak – is recognized only when it is too late, i.e., when the patient has already developed diffuse peritonitis. In up to 60% of cases, postoperative peritonitis results in patient death [379]. It is also important to assess secretions from the drain on the basis of smell and color. For deep colorectal or coloanal anastomoses, a leak may be diagnosed by simple digital or endoscopic examination. A conservative approach may be chosen for small leaks, with a correctly placed drain that can remove the inflammatory exudate from the body. More extensive leaks, if located extraperitoneal in the pelvis minor, may heal without suturing, if a protective stoma is placed in order to relieve the bowel [380]. If ultrasound sonography shows presence of free fluid in the abdomen, if an abscess cannot be drained, or when faced with the early stages of peritonitis, surgery must be indicated as early as possible. If the leak is small and only recently developed, closing the gap with a protective stoma may be considered [381]. As in the past, discontinuity resection is the standard procedure, if diffuse peritonitis develops. In case of an anastomotic leak, the surgical strategy is determined primarily by the clinical condition of the patient. As early as the 70s of the previous century, Goligher et al. [382] showed that of the 60% of leaks that could be radiologically detected, after deep anterior resection only 25% manifested itself clinically at all.

For several years now, the principle behind vacuum assisted therapy, which is used to treat poorly healing wounds, is also applied to healing of the inner surface of the colon. Vacuum therapy unifies three therapeutic principles: the infection is kept under control locally, due to stimulation of the granulation process, the wound size is reduced, and the healing process is geared towards the specific nature of the colonic lumen. For deep anastomotic leaks, the healing process can be controlled proctoscopically, under vision [383].

Among the overwhelming amount of medical malpractice claims associated with anastomotic leaks, the majority involves suspected or actual deficiencies in the management of complications. Typically, the defendant is accused of reacting to symptoms indicating a leak either too late, or inadequately, or even of not reacting at all.

The development of an anastomotic leak does not as such create any liability issues, but rather the question of how they are treated and whether any problems are recognized timely enough.

Hence, the key to successful management of these types of complications and successful defense against malpractice claims lies in rapid and targeted diagnostics and - most of all – in "paying attention".

2.7.7 Examples of liability issues

Example 1
Laparoscopic-assisted sigmoid resection (descendo-rectostomy), using the double-stapling technique, was performed on a 57-year-old patient, with recurrent sigmoid

diverticulitis. No abnormal postoperative increase of body temperature was noted. The first bowel passage was on the third day post-op. On the fifth day post-op, complaints about abdominal pain appeared, for which the patient was given an analgesic. A bloated abdomen was seen, but no extensive examination was conducted. An ultrasound scan did not show any free abdominal fluid, but the patient's bladder was seen to be full. The bladder was drained via catheterization. Furthermore, the inflammatory parameters started to increase dramatically. Two days later, a contrast CT scan of the abdomen was conducted, showing large amounts of free intraabdominal fluid. This was followed by an endoscopic examination, in which an extended perforation, close to and above the anastomosis, was found. The ensuing laparotomy verified an anastomotic leak, affecting two-thirds of the circumference of the bowel. Additionally, diffuse peritonitis was found, with ubiquitous prior fibrin deposits on the intestinal loops. Discontinuity resection was performed, and a terminal descendostomy was created. The abdomen was provisionally closed, pending a second-look operation. After surgery, the patient had to be treated in ICU for four weeks, due to severe sepsis and multiple organ failure. In the further course of treatment, four planned revision laparotomies were conducted. After a final sanitation of the diffuse peritonitis, the abdomen could be permanently closed.

Conclusion: On the fifth day post-op, the patient's condition - which so far had been nondescript - worsened, with development of acute abdominal pain and a bloated stomach. On the basis of these symptoms, targeted examinations, e.g., endoscopy or contrast CT with a water-soluble contrast agent should have been conducted immediately. Relaparotomy was delayed for at least two days, despite development of peritonitis, leading to an extended stay in ICU and multiple revision operations.

Example 2
A 39-year-old male underwent laparoscopically assisted sigmoid resection to treat perforated sigmoid diverticulitis. The anamnesis mentioned excessive alcohol and nicotine abuse. Early postoperative progression was normal, and the patient rapidly regained his mobility. As early as the first day post-op, the patient was able to move around, and he mentioned only minor pain. On the 5th day, the patient started to complain about sharp and increasingly intense abdominal pain. The intra-abdominal drain, through which only very small amounts of secretions had been discharged so far, was removed. On the 6th day post-op, tachycardia developed and the patient began to suffer attacks of severe perspiration. He became restless and delirious, which was attributed to withdrawal effects from his alcohol and nicotine abuse. On the 7th day post-op, the patient collapsed. Fecal secretion was seen to discharge from the previous location of the drain. Up to that, no clinical findings had been documented. Emergency laparotomy on the 7th day post-op found peritonitis, caused by an anastomotic leak. During the ensuing discontinuity resection after Hartmann, the affected tissue was removed, the abdomen lavaged and left open (called "open packing"), in light of further planned revision laparotomies. The patient was mechanically ventilated on ICU for five weeks, and intermittent hemodialysis was necessary, due to renal failure.

Conclusion: The decreased level of awareness, akathisia, and delirium, accompanied by fever and tachycardia, were assessed to be withdrawal effects from alcohol and drugs. However, such symptoms are equally likely to be a clinical manifestation of an anastomotic leak. A differential diagnosis should have been made to determine whether the patient's worsening condition might be attributed to something more harmful, i.e., an anastomotic leak with ensuing peritonitis.

Hence, in this case, the fundamental standard of due diligence was violated. The management of complications, as well as the diagnostics and documentation of clinical findings, was deficient.

Example 3

A 70-year-old female patient with rectal prolapse underwent laparoscopic-assisted rectopexy and a transanal, double-stapled anastomosis was performed. According to the OR report, both mucosal rings were found intact and circular in shape. Anastomotic sealing was checked by air insufflation and lavaging. After increasing abdominal pain, an X-ray examination was conducted on the 3rd day post-op, which showed evidence of anastomotic leakage. The ensuing relaparoscopy confirmed presence of an extensive leak, caused by incomplete closure of the stapled seam. The staples were not closed into typical "B" shape, but still retained their original shape, over a distance of 3 cm.

Conclusion: This particular anastomotic leak was caused by malfunction of the stapler.

The department of the German Federal Institute for Drugs and Medical Devices (BfArM) responsible for medical equipment records any reported incidents in light of § 2 and § 3 of the Medical Devices Safety Plan Ordinance (MPSV). Barth [384] and others evaluated incidents with surgical stapling devices, reported to the BfArM from 2002 to 2007. The most frequently occurring error patterns were: "device is empty or did not release its staples ..." or: "staples not closing properly, seam or anastomosis incomplete ...", " instrument could not be opened and cartridge could not be removed after staples were released ...", "cutting function was actuated, but seam was created incorrectly or not at all ...". During the above period, a total number of 165 incidents, involving the above error patterns, were registered.

A total of 58 reports mentioned patient injuries, part of them severe. In 45 incidents (27%), with varying characteristics, examination by the manufacturer confirmed product defect, upon which corrective measures were taken. In 52.73% of cases, the manufacturer could not find any defects in the returned instruments.

2.7.8 Summary

Anastomotic leaks in the upper and lower gastrointestinal tract are associated with high morbidity and mortality rates.

Early diagnosis and treatment, in conjunction with management of complications guided by the clinical findings, are decisive for the outcome. Belated diagnostics and delayed treatment of an anastomotic leak, in particular, may give rise to malpractice claims.

2.8 Diagnostic and therapeutical errors in the treatment of acute abdomen

2.8.1 Introduction

The term "acute abdomen", or "undifferentiated abdominal pain" (UDAP), does not denote a specific disease, but rather describes a conglomerate of symptoms involving acute, or acutely recurrent, abdominal pain, with a peritoneal component. Hence, "acute abdomen" is a working diagnosis. Its leading symptoms are, e.g., severe, acute abdominal pain or peritoneal irritation, often in conjunction with disruption of normal bowel peristalsis. This working diagnosis demands immediate action. Targeted anamnesis, thorough clinical examinations and observation, are used to make a differential diagnosis, which is completed by laboratory tests and diagnostic imaging. Diagnosing this often life-threatening condition requires a large amount of technical experience and commands close cooperation between multiple medical specialties. Misassessment, incomplete and belated diagnostics, as well as delayed and incorrect indication for surgery, often lead to liability claims.

2.8.2 Fundamentals

Surgical textbooks describe more than 70 possible underlying diseases capable of causing acute abdomen [385] which may be determined through a differential diagnosis. For example:

Tab. 2.7: Causes of acute abdomen [386–388]

Cause	Frequency
Atypical abdominal pain	33%
Appendicitis	28%
Cholecystitis	10%
Mechanical ileus	4%
Acute gynecological diseases (extrauterine gravidity, adnexitis)	4%
Pancreatitis	3%
Renal colic	3%
Perforated ulcer	3%
Diverticulitis	2%
Peritonitis	Rare
Testicular torsion (esp. in children and young adults)	Rare
Ischemic bowel disease (esp. in geriatric patients, mesenteric infarction, ischemic colitis)	Rare
Splenic infarction	Rare
Ruptured spleen, liver or kidney	Rare
Internal bleeding (retroperitoneal, m. rectus abdominis)	Rare
Surgical complications (seam failure, infected hematoma, peritonitis, abscess)	Rare
Fulminant clostridium difficile colitis	Rare

A study conducted by the World Gastroenterology Organization (OMGE - Organisation Mondiale de Gastro-Entérologie) [389] shows that two thirds of cases of acute abdomen are caused by atypical abdominal pain, acute appendicitis, or acute cholecystitis.

Myocardial infarction, acute coronary syndrome, pericarditis, pulmonary embolism, basal pneumonitis, pneumothorax, but also spinal disorders are possible extra-abdominal causes of acute abdomen. The possibility of an intestinal pseudo-obstruction must also be factored into the differential diagnosis, as well as metabolic disorders such as lactic acidosis, diabetic ketoacidosis, and others. Due to the plethora of possible differential diagnoses, treatment must often be initiated before the actual cause of the symptoms has been found. Potentially fatal conditions, such as myocardial infarction, ruptured or symptomatic aortic aneurysm, acute mesenteric ischemia, and ectopic pregnancy or a ruptured fallopian tube, may also cause acute abdomen. If any of these diseases has caused the acute abdomen, misdiagnosis may have fatal consequences. Immediate surgery is indicated in case of, e.g., acute bleeding. A perforated hollow viscus, mesenteric infarction, or diffuse peritonitis, require emergency surgery (within less than two hours). Urgent surgery (within less than eight hours) is indicated for acute appendicitis, perforated sigmoid diverticulitis, or toxic megacolon. Assessment of the patient's general clinical condition, but especially presence of diffuse muscular defense, determined by an experienced physician, guides the clinician to deciding whether surgery is indicated [390]. If a situation requires immediate action, the clinician must decide if conservative observation in conjunction with pharmacotherapy may be justified. In this case, the clinical condition of the patient must be monitored at regular intervals, and all findings, must be documented in the medical case file, including timestamps. In this critical phase, incorrect or missing documentation or failure to scrutinize findings that, from a professional point of view, require close examination may substantiate malpractice claims. Special vigilance is required when treating high-risk patients - usually elderly people whose immune system has been compromised. In such patients, clinical symptoms frequently come in disguise and manifest themselves less obviously. For example, in elderly patients, presence of muscular defense - the leading symptom of a burst appendix - often manifests itself less distinctively or not at all, despite presence of peritonitis or a perityphlitic abscess. It is important to make a detailed and targeted anamnesis, so that signs of prior diseases, capable of causing acute abdomen, may be detected. It is also important to record the patient's medication history, for example, an existing peptic ulcer or chronic pancreatitis in connection with alcoholism. The anamnesis can, however, also steer the physician towards a misdiagnosis, for example, if the patient's history includes recurrent gallstones, but the present symptoms are actually due to myocardial infarction. In this case, it may have fatal consequences if the patient is misdiagnosed with cholecystitis and cholecystectomy is performed, although in reality the symptoms are caused by a myocardial infarction! A particularly tricky case is the so-called painless acute abdomen - the painless interval after initially very intense acute pain. This pattern often occurs with intestinal perforations or a perforated hollow viscus and can lure the physician into a false sense of security. Although possibly life-threatening, gastrointestinal bleeding often does not cause pain and manifests itself with only mild symptoms. An abdominal X-ray scan may show a perforation, presence of a foreign body, or signs typical of ileus. However, conventional X-ray examinations find relevant results in only ca. 7% of cases. In contrast, a sonographic exam may be conducted rapidly and immediately, at the patient's bedside. It rates high for detecting free abdominal fluid, and immediate paracentesis to drain it off may be safely performed. As described above, prospective studies on ultrasound diagnosis with acute appendicitis show 72–90% sensitivity and 92–100% specificity [391]. However, in one third of cases, it cannot successfully diagnose acute appendicitis [392], in contrast with an abdominal CT scan, which has 90.1% sensitivity and 94.1% specificity to acute appendicitis [393].

Even if sonographic or CT evidence shows no abnormalities, it may still not be possible to unambiguously indicate or contraindicate surgery in individual cases. For individual cases of acute abdomen, Pathways or Sore-systems are not sufficient to determine a definitive course of action or to guide differential diagnostics, as exemplified by the still rather high rate of burst appendices, despite close inpatient observation, which, surprisingly, hardly changed during the last 70 years, still ranging between 20 and 30% [394]. In addition, due to the immense complexity of acute abdomen, close interdisciplinary cooperation between surgeons and, depending on the occasion, urologists, internists, gynecologists, and radiologists is mandated. In case of doubt, if the clinical situation remains unclear, the physician should opt for surgery. A negative laparotomy/laparoscopy, meaning that no pathologies are found, generally does not substantiate malpractice claims. The following quote applies to all undetermined cases:

> "In doubtful cases do not wait too long,
> Before exploring for it is quite wrong
> To act upon the slogan wait and see
> When looking might provide the remedy." [395]

"A negative relaparotomy is better than a positive autopsy but is not, nevertheless, a benign procedure" [396].

We will now discuss some examples of surgical diseases, for which alleged or actual errors in disease management frequently lead to malpractice claims. In particular:

1. Diffuse peritonitis
2. Ileus
3. Mesenteric ischemia

2.8.3 Malpractice claims and complications related to peritonitis and abdominal sepsis

2.8.3.1 Peritonitis with abdominal sepsis

With 20%, the mortality rate as a result of severe intraabdominal infections remains very high, despite progress in surgical technology and improvements in intensive care medicine [397–403]. Primary peritonitis involves hematogenous, lymphogenic, or intraluminal infections in the peritoneal cavity. Hence, primary peritonitis is largely the domain of conservative therapy. Secondary peritonitis, caused by injuries to the hollow viscera in the vicinity of the gastrointestinal tract, falls under the domain of surgery. If peritonitis persists or recurs, despite adequate surgery, antimicrobial treatment, and intensive therapy, this is classified as tertiary peritonitis.

Postoperative peritonitis after abdominal surgery, lethal in up to 60% of cases, is a special case of secondary peritonitis [404, 405].

In 2001, the International Sepsis Definitions Conference, represented by, a.o., the Society of Critical Care Medicine (SCCM), the European Society of Intensive Care Medicine (ESICM), and the Surgical Infection Society (SIS), redefined the notion of "systemic inflammatory response to infection" [406].

In the past, multiple scoring systems were suggested for risk assessment in cases of abdominal sepsis.

The APACHE-II score for general risk assessment in ICU patients has been widely accepted. The Acute Physiology and Chronic Health Evaluation (APACHE) II score [407], Multiple Organ Dysfunction Score (MODS) [408], and the Sepsis-related Organ Functional Assessment (SOFA) score [409] reflect the correlation between severity of the disease and the associated mortality rate.

Treatment of abdominal sepsis rests on three elementary therapeutic pillars:

1. Surgical sanitation of the source of the infection
2. Systemic antimicrobial therapy
3. ICU treatment of septic organ failure

Decisive prognostic factors are to determine the diagnosis as soon as possible and to immediately initiate treatment. During initial revision surgery, the surgeon should target rigorous sanitation of the source of the infection, which is a key step in the procedure. The rate of mortality is correlated with successful sanitization of the initial inflammatory source and elimination of bacteria and toxins from the abdominal cavity [410, 411]. Many clinics perform discontinuity resection to treat perforated sigmoid diverticulitis stadium III and IV after Hinchey. However, based on experiences with first-track surgery, a substantial amount of authors prefer resection of the affected intestinal segment and performing a primary anastomosis over a Hartmann operation, because the latter carries a significantly higher mortality risk [412]. If bowel ischemia is caused by vascular factors, resection of the infarcted intestinal segments is performed, frequently followed by discontinuity resection. During a second look operation one or two days later, the blood supply to the remaining colon can be assessed and an anastomosis can be performed, should this be necessary. There exist a large number of additive concepts that help prevent persisting or recurring peritonitis after successful sanitation of the inflamed area: abundant lavaging of the abdominal cavity dilutes the amount of remaining bacteria and helps support the organism's immunity system. So far, however, this idea that lavaging and dilution does in fact quantitatively remove bacteria from the peritoneal surface has not been supported by conclusive evidence [413]. Between 1970 and 1980, numerous additive concepts for treatment of peritonitis were established, for example, continuous postoperative lavage [414, 415], planned postoperative relaparotomy [416–419], or the so-called open abdomen [420]. A primary laparostomy (open packing) is supposed to relieve high intraabdominal pressure and to facilitate improved mesenteric circulation and ventilation. A disadvantage of this method is the comparatively high associated mortality rate. According to a recent study, ca. 50% of patients develop multiple organ failure after creation of a laparostoma. For 48%, severe bleeding or secondary fistulas developed [421]. The situation is aggravated by additional contamination of the abdominal cavity with exogenous bacteria. Hence, many surgeons have abandoned the principle of a primary open abdomen [417, 422]. If the source of the infection is thoroughly sanitized, a single operation is sufficient in 90% of cases [423]. The concept of "relaparotomy on demand" (RoD) aims to conduct relaparotomy only if the clinical situation does not improve or worsens. A meta-analysis, comprising eight studies, which compared RoD with so-called programmed lavage, showed a non-significant advantage for RoD [424]. However, a significant advantage over programmed lavage was found in another retrospective analysis that involved 278 patients with secondary peritonitis [425]. Urgent relaparotomy is indicated, if the abdomen is exposed, if the drain contains fecal matter, or if an abdominal compartment syndrome threatens to develop. An intra-abdominal pressure of more than 22 mmHg is as an absolute indication for surgical decompression. If an intra-abdominal compartment syndrome has developed, the associated mortality rate can be up to 50% [426].

Most malpractice claims in relation to peritonitis do not concern its cause, but rather what is judged to be deficient complication management.

2.8.4 Real-life examples

Example 1
A 33-year-old female patient with acute abdomen was admitted to hospital. Examination upon admission found diffuse abdominal pressure pain, with punctum maximum in the left lower abdomen. No free air was seen in the X-ray scan. An ultrasound scan showed severe coprostasis. Initially, inflammatory parameters were strongly elevated. On the next day, a severe decrease in white blood cell count, at only 1,100 leukocytes/µl. Additional decrease in thrombocyte count and coagulation factors, with simultaneous increase of renal retention parameters into the pathological range, indicating renal failure. Laparotomy was performed only the next day. A perforated sigmoid colon was found, caused by an impacted fecaloma, leading to diffuse peritonitis. Postoperatively, the patient was transferred to a university clinic, with clear signs of a Systemic Inflammatory Response Syndrome (SIRS). Diffuse peritonitis necessitated five relaparotomies. The patient suffered prolonged sepsis with multiple organ failure, and needed continuous mandatory ventilation for 15 days.

Conclusion: Delayed relaparotomy in an already advanced state of peritonitis.

Example 2
A 55-year-old male patient suffered blunt abdominal trauma when, at work, a 500 kg steel pipe impacted the ventral abdominal wall. On admission to hospital, an extended supraumbilical hematoma was noted. An abdominal ultrasound scan did not show any free abdominal fluid. Laboratory tests did not indicate anemia. Distinctive leukocytosis was noted, at 18,000/µl. Amylase, lipase, lactate, and LDH were not determined. Eight hours after admission, a renewed laboratory test established thrombocytopenia and leukocytopenia. A second ultrasound examination now showed free abdominal fluid. Fourteen hours after admission, laparotomy was performed, and a 2 cm long rupture in the sigmoid colon wall was found, together with multiple serosal lesions near both sigmoid and descending colon. The rupture site was oversewn. Postoperatively, the patient was further treated in ICU, where sepsis developed, in conjunction with high fever and circulatory depression, which had to be treated with high doses of catecholamines. Furthermore, the patient developed severe metabolic acidosis. Laboratory tests established leukocytopenia with a white blood cell count of 1,300–1,000/µl, a continuous increase of CRP values, and a rapid decrease of coagulation factors. On the second day post-op, the patient was transferred to a university clinic and immediately underwent relaparotomy. During surgery, a preexisting diffuse peritonitis was found, emanating from a pea-sized perforation in the terminal ileum, which had been excised and oversewn.

Conclusion: Blunt abdominal trauma had perforated the bowel in two places. Only the perforation in the sigmoid bowel had been treated in the first operation. The second, smaller perforation in the terminal ileum, which had caused the diffuse peritonitis, had been erroneously overlooked. Relaparotomy had been indicated belatedly.

Example 3

A 58-year-old female patient underwent colonoscopy, after complaining of bloody discharge through the rectum. Endoscopic findings noted that, during the examination, an atypical, strongly swollen abdomen developed, but found questionable indication of a sigmoid colon perforation. Immediately after the endoscopy, the patient was transferred to the nearest major hospital. During transport, the bulging abdomen stood under maximum pressure. At 77%, oxygen saturation was severely reduced. On admission, both legs showed a distinct, mottled, bluish discoloration. During relaparotomy, more than three hours after admission, large quantities of free air escaped from the abdomen. A 4 cm long perforation was found in the middle part of the sigmoid colon and was oversewn. Strong intraoperative tendency to diffuse bleeding. Laboratory tests confirmed a severe decrease of coagulation factors, with AT III having dropped to 25%. On admission to ICU, cardiovascular circulation became unstable. Laboratory tests showed severe lactic acidosis. The tendency to diffuse bleeding necessitated massive blood and coagulation factors transfusions. The patient was resuscitated twice but died from irreversible septic-toxic circulatory failure two days after being admitted.

Conclusion: During colonoscopy tension pneumoperitoneum had developed, and the colon was perforated, leading to development of the abdominal compartment syndrome. Here, the fact that the visibly increased intra-abdominal pressure was not immediately relieved was a culpable error. The increased pressure had caused compression of the a. and v. cava, leading to ischemia in both legs. The restricted blood flow through the venae cavae back to the heart finally caused circulatory shock. On admission to the hospital, this acute, life-threatening situation should already have been obvious to the attending physicians. The tension pneumoperitoneum should have been relieved immediately upon admission.

Example 4

Due to tachycardia and sudden attacks of perspiration, a 52-year-old patient was admitted to hospital for inpatient treatment. A stomach ulcer had been known to exist for 25 years. Basic laboratory tests on admission showed no abnormalities. X-ray examination, clinical observation, or abdominal ultrasound examination was not performed. The patient was given an analgesic to treat the symptoms. Due to persisting abdominal pain, a conventional abdominal X-ray exam was conducted, but no free air could be seen. However, an ultrasound scan showed larger amounts of free abdominal fluid. Laparotomy was performed 30 hours after admission, as indicated by acute abdomen. The laparotomy confirmed diffuse peritonitis, emanating from a perforated prepyloric ulcer. Protracted circulatory depression was noted intraoperatively. The stomach ulcer was excised, and the wound was sutured. Shortly after transfer to ICU, the patient went into cardiac arrest and was hypoxic for an extended period. After resuscitation, permanent brain damage due to a midbrain symptom.

Conclusion: The patient, suffering from a known stomach ulcer, was admitted for inpatient treatment with tachycardia, sudden attacks of perspiration, and strong epigastric pain. No targeted clinical examinations were conducted on initial admission or during further treatment. The attending physicians should have realized that free air in the abdomen is seen on X-ray scans in only ca. 70% of cases. Hence, lack of radiological evidence of free air in no way excludes the presence of a perforation. Although mandatorily indicated on admission, laparotomy was performed with a delay of at least 24 hours, after diffuse peritonitis had already developed. The septic-toxic cardiac arrest could be explained by toxins generated by the peritonitis entering the bloodstream, with circulatory collapse and hypoxic brain damage as dramatic consequences.

2.8.5 Ileus

A rough distinction may be made between mechanical and paralytic ileus. Mechanical ileus is caused by constriction of the intestinal passage due to adhesions and adhesive strands - with or without bending or torqueing of the bowel - by inflammatory or tumorous stenosis, gallstones, feces, worms, or other factors. Incarceration, invagination, or volvulus can lead to reduced mesenteric blood supply. In a paralytic ileus, the intestinal motility is paralyzed due to, for example, intraabdominal inflammations and infections, or due to mesenteric vein thrombosis, arterial embolism in the a. mesenterica superior, the non-occlusive disease, various forms of vasculitis, but also due to various metabolic diseases such as diabetic acidosis. Paralytic ileus may also be caused by some classes of pharmaceuticals, including opiates and antidepressants. Of particular relevance to our discussion is the postoperative ileus. The transition from regular postoperative bowel atony to true ileus may be very gradual, which hampers diagnostics. Strangulation ileus is a special case of mechanical ileus, since the strangulation mechanism may cause early disruption or restriction of mesenteric blood supply. Consequently, besides mechanical obstruction, rapid ischemic damage is done to the mucous membranes, which then ceases to be a barrier to bacteria and toxins. In such cases, the risk of developing transmigration peritonitis or a perforation of the strangulated intestinal segment inside the abdominal cavity is exceptionally high [427]. Depending on location, an obstruction may initiate various different pathophysiological events, thus motivating a classification that discriminates between large intestine ileus (20–25% of these types of disorders) and small intestine ileus (75–80%). The latter can be further divided into high and deep small intestine ileus. Deep ileus is characterized most of all by rapid multiplication of toxin forming fecal bacteria. The high toxin concentration enables endotoxins, released by gram-negative bacteria, to penetrate the intestinal wall and trigger a complex cascade of inflammatory processes, such as induction of lipoxigenase and cyclooxigenases activity and stimulation of thromboxane and prostaglandin synthesis. The bowels contain the largest organ of immunity within the human body (Gut Associated Lymphatic Tissue, GALT) and accommodate more than half of its total number of granulocytes. Leaks in the gastric mucous barrier facilitate bacterial translocation and cause systemic effects that may trigger the Systemic Inflammatory Response Syndrome (SIRS) or lead to multiple organ failure. Other mediators that are released (histamine, serotonin, bradykinin), interact with toxins to paralyze the bowel's smooth muscle tissue [428–431]. Full-blown ileus is characterized by hypovolemia, absorption of endotoxins by the bowel, and organ failure. In small intestine ileus, the obstruction is often located in the jejunum [432]. A dangerous and rather typical aspect of the situation just described, is pronounced reflux of stomach and bowel secretions, with consecutive rapid disruption of electrolyte balance, typified most of all by violent vomiting. Usually, X-ray and ultrasound findings appear inconspicuous, because there is no distention of the stomach or other bowel segments. In contrast to deep ileus, no mediators are released. On the other hand, disruptions in the organism's fluid and electrolyte balance become prominent, and must be counteracted with (if necessary intravenous) substitution therapy.

It is critically important for successful treatment to recognize ileus and correctly determine its degree of severity. As mentioned earlier, during further treatment, true ileus must be distinguished from a physiological post-operative paralysis. The anamnesis plays a central role within the diagnostic algorithm, along with (possibly repeated) subtle clinical examinations. Diagnostics is completed with medical imaging and laboratory tests. During anamnesis the clinician documents any prior or existing diseases, and, if applicable, prior operations. Clinical symptoms come in a large variety, with patients often complaining of colicky pain, nausea, and vomiting, as well as inability to defecate. Patients that suffer a high ileus may report "normal" bowel movement. In contrast, in case of deep ileus, vomiting and nausea are often absent. Presence of peritonitis or muscular defense usually is the exception and only occurs after the bowel has been ruptured and peritonitis has developed. The presence of ileus or of intestinal incarcerations cannot be exclusively determined or excluded by laboratory tests. Nevertheless, these tests are an important component of the diagnostic work-up, since disruptions of electrolyte balance, dehydration, and elevated inflammation parameters may provide valuable clues to the severity of the disease. Lactate testing may reveal impaired blood supply to one or more bowel segments. However, in case of simultaneous arterial and venous occlusion, the lactate concentration in the peripheral blood need not be elevated. Renzulli et al. [433] were able to show that leukocytosis and fever higher than 37.8°C occurred for only 67% of patients with a clinically manifesting ileus. Tachycardia was present in 65%. Only 71% reported local pressure pain. In cases where intestinal necrosis had developed, only 29% suffered pressure pain and in only 26% of cases leukocytosis or elevated temperature developed.

The decision for surgery can only be made after reviewing the complete picture, consisting of anamnesis, clinical examination, medical imaging, and laboratory tests. Conventional X-ray exams often cannot discriminate between small intestine and large intestine ileus. In case of ileus due to a gallstone, free air can typically be seen in the bile ducts. An ultrasound scan can verify dilated intestinal loops, bowel wall thickening, free abdominal fluid and other pathologies that accompany ileus. In case of large intestine ileus, an enema with a water-soluble contrast agent and ensuing CT scan may be a helpful next step.

Ileus is responsible for ca. 4% of all laparotomies conducted in surgical clinics. Ca. 70% are in the small intestine. Ca. 20% of admissions with acute abdomen are caused by small intestine ileus [434]. Due to the increasing incidence of abdominal surgery, the most frequent causes of small intestine ileus are adhesions and adhesive bands [435–437]. Opening the peritoneal cavity leads to formation of potentially obstructive structures (adhesions or adhesive bands) in almost 95% of patients [438]. After adhesive ileus surgery, the risk of developing another mechanical ileus within three years post-op lies between 8.7% and 53% [435, 439–442].

If strangulation or bowel ischemia is suspected, surgery is absolutely indicated for all forms of ileus, with no further need to find unambiguous parameters with definitive predictive power. If there are no clues that may lead the physician to suspect a disrupted blood flow, conservative treatment with parenteral fluid substitution or intestinal tube decompression may be tried [443]. However, even if the dilated bowel is relieved with a tube or in some cases even through normal defecation, it may not be concluded that ileus is no longer present! If the cause is visible from the outside, for instance, in case of an incarcerated inguinal hernia, the indication for surgery is self-evident. Today, the prior requirement to perform early surgery on principle, in case of total blockage due to mechanical ileus, has only limited validity. As long as the patient's condition justifies it, a delay of 48 hours or, in exceptional cases, up to five days is considered reasonable [444]. In each individual case, the potential risks and disadvantages of laparotomy, such as renewed formation of adhesions, must be weighed against the possibility of an unnoticed ischemia or against possible rectification of the causes of the ileus. The risks connected with tube decompression are due to the immoderate expansion of its indications to include even complete bowel obstructions, for which the chances of successful relief are rather small [445–448]. Eliminating the cause of the ileus and restoring natural intestinal transport function are the primary therapeutic targets. If a single adhesion is present, it may be sufficient to sever it surgically. In case of extensive adhesions, complete adhesiolysis becomes necessary. If the obstruction is due to a tumor, the surgical procedure is determined by the clinical findings. If possible, the physician should aim at primary resection of intestinal segments. Usually, if there is a pronounced infestation of the tumor into the pelvis and the lower abdomen, the only remaining option is to create an ileostomy. If the ileus is not operated immediately after inpatient admission, the patient must be monitored by conducting fine-grained clinical examinations, laboratory tests, and (occasionally) medical imaging. In general, it can be determined if surgery is or might become necessary within the first 24 hours. If the ileus is suspected to be due to a single adhesive band, and if the patient underwent no extensive prior surgery, diagnostic laparoscopy may be considered [449, 450].

Stenosing tumors are a frequent cause of large intestine ileus. In case of a stenosing rectal tumor, it must be determined if state of the art radiochemotherapy may be initially indicated. If a perforation with accompanying peritonitis developed, the physician should not hesitate to indicate bowel resection with creation of a stoma [451].

2.8.6 Malpractice claims related to surgical ileus treatment

As a rule, malpractice claims arising from the ileus treatment do not concern the surgical aspect, but rather involve preoperative and postoperative disease management. In most cases, the defendant is accused of not displaying medical due diligence during examination and diagnosis and a belated indication for surgery.

2.8.7 Real-life examples

Example 1
A 78-year-old female patient was admitted to hospital after persistent vomiting, starting two weeks prior to admission. Laboratory findings showed pronounced

elevation of the inflammation parameters. Clinical examination found the abdomen tender, without isolated pressure pain. No pathological resistance was felt. Ultrasound examination led to the suspicion of a gallstone. A conventional abdominal X-ray scan showed accumulation of fluid in multiple places, thus pointing towards small intestine ileus. A stomach tube was inserted to relieve the patient. A CT scan, conducted on the third day, showed multiple adhesions in the small and large intestines. On the eighth day after inpatient admission, due to lack of clinical improvement, laparotomy was performed. During surgery, massive discharge of small intestine content through a perforation in the terminal ileum, right before the ileocecal valve. The perforation was caused by a blocking gallstone, which had caused gallstone ileus with ensuing intestinal perforation and development of peritonitis. Reexamination of the original X-ray images uncovered multiple air bubbles in the bile ducts.

Conclusion: Gallstone ileus should have been noticed immediately if the clinician had displayed due diligence when interpreting the X-ray images, but was overlooked.

An estimated two to four out of every 1,000 patients with cholelithiasis develop gallstone ileus [452]. The anamnesis can take hours to weeks, and rather frequently findings are uncharacteristic. In many cases, the clinical image is that of a "whimsical, sloppy" ileus [453].

Example 2
A 48-year-old female patient, without prior abdominal surgery, was admitted to the emergency room with complaints of extreme abdominal pain after eating. The abdominal surface was examined, and the abdominal wall was found tender and tension-free. Abdominal auscultation was not performed or not documented. Ultrasound examination was not possible, due to the patient's restlessness and extreme spasmodic abdominal pain. Laboratory test showed elevated inflammation parameters, including the lactic acid value. The patient was treated symptomatically with an analgesic. However, she kept complaining about increasingly intense colicky pain and suffered multiple surges of vomiting.

A laboratory test on the next day, ca. 20 hours after admission, showed a massively increased white blood cell count and lactic acid value. Under the assumption of a gynecological disease, a transvaginal ultrasound examination was conducted, which showed larger amounts of free abdominal fluid in the recto-uterine pouch. More than 30 hours after admission, laparotomy was conducted and found massive small intestine ileus, caused by a mobile megacecum with complete volvulus of the caecum and the small intestine, wrapped 360° around the small bowel mesentery. In the ileum and in larger segments of the jejunum, ischemic necrosis had developed. Only 1.5 m of the jejunum had a sufficient blood supply, and could be saved. Due to a postoperative short bowel syndrome, a Hickman line had to be placed.

Conclusion: In light of the dramatic symptoms, which, given the elevated lactic acid value, should make one strongly suspect ileus, emergency surgery should have been indicated in an earlier stage. Primary diagnostics and further observation during inpatient treatment were deficient and not appropriate to the severity of the disease.

Example 3

A 56-year-old patient underwent right hemicolectomy to treat a ca. 4 cm long tubulovillous adenoma. Starting on the third day post-op, increased meteorism, regular vomiting and strongly elevated CRP levels were noted. Vomiting became more frequent from the fourth day post-op, and the patient developed more than 38.2°C fever. Late in the evening of the fourth day post-op, a gastric tube was placed, through which 2,400 ml gastric and small intestine content surged out immediately. On the fifth day post-op, further massive elevation of the inflammation parameters. On the sixth day post-op a CT scan was made, which showed a large amount of free abdominal fluid and massively dilated small bowel loops. By now, the renal retention parameters also were elevated, with reduced diuresis. On the seventh day post-op, the clinical pattern belonging to full-blown anuria emerged, in conjunction with increasing circulatory lability. In the early morning of the eighth day post-op, the patient was found dead in bed. The patient's relatives refused autopsy on religious grounds.

Conclusion: Surgical intervention was deferred, despite classical symptoms of postoperative small intestine ileus. In light of the patient's life-threatening condition, including high fever, circulatory lability, and early symptoms of shock, it was - from a professional point of view - incomprehensible, that transfer to an ICU had not been expedited and surgery was not performed at an earlier time. A similar lack of comprehension applies to the failure to conduct fine-grained clinical and laboratory tests, despite presence of classical symptoms of ileus.

2.8.8 Mesenteric ischemia

2.8.8.1 Diagnostic and therapeutic errors related to mesenteric ischemia

If a high-risk patient consults a physician and complains about abdominal pain persisting for more than two or three hours, which cannot be attributed to any immediate cause, AGA guidelines (American Gastroenterological Association, AGA 2000) recommend to check for possible mesenteric ischemia. Patients over 50 years old and/or suffering from cardiac insufficiency, cardiac arrhythmia, myocardial infarction in the recent past, hypervolemia, hypotonia, or sepsis are considered to be especially at risk [454]. The following quotation applies:

"... For a patient with mesenteric ischemia, the prognosis critically depends on the steps taken by the physician who conducts the initial examination. Rapid, targeted, and - frequently enough - invasive and aggressive diagnostics, in conjunction with the ensuing therapy can save lives; Wait-and-see approaches that rely on close monitoring and controlling almost always result in patient death. Pathological laboratory values such as leukocytosis, metabolic acidosis or elevated lactate value are arguments that mandate mesenteric angiography, which is the gold standard for determining presence of arterial mesenteric ischemia ..." [454].

It is a known fact that, for patients over 80 years of age, the chance of so-called "acute abdomen" being due to mesenteric ischemia is many times higher than for younger patients [455]. The de facto incidence of mesenteric ischemia as cause of acute abdomen may be even larger, because 60% of all mesenteric infarctions are diagnosed post mortem [456, 457]. If left untreated an acute arterial mesenteric infarction is lethal in 80–100% of cases. For untreated mesenteric venous thrombosis, the mortality rate is 50% [455].

It may be considered as given, that the time interval between onset of symptoms and initiation of treatment has a decisive influence on the patient's prognosis [455]. Villous atrophy occurs as little as 30 minutes after onset of total ischemia. After more than 60 minutes, hypoxic damage to the tunica muscularis and, at a later stage, the tunica serosa may be expected.

Numerous studies have shown that any time lost in the clinic is associated with a significantly increased mortality rate, as can be seen in the following table.

Tab. 2.8: Influence of the time interval between onset of symptoms and determination of the diagnosis/initiation of therapy on the mortality rate of acute mesenteric ischemia

Author	N	< 12 h	12–24 h	> 24 h
Boley et al. [458]	47	–	57%	73%
Ritz et al. [459]	141	17%	61%	92%
Walter et al. [460]	46	36%	63%	95%
Paes et al. [461]	–	33%	62%	79%
Inderbitzi et al. a) [462]	26	0%	58%	88%
Bjorck et al. b) [463]	60	40%	67% (> 12 h)	

a) Patients underwent embolectomy and/or bowel resection.
b) Time between onset of symptoms and initial clinical examination.

In addition, it must be kept in mind that the likelihood of total mesenteric infarction increases as the patient gets older. Hence, for elderly patients, the time factor is especially important. The group led by Ritz [459], for example, pointed out that the increased mortality rate for older patients is mainly due to delays in inpatient admission and that they have a higher chance of survival if surgery is performed at an early stage [459, 464].

2.8.9 Real-life example

Example 1
An 81-year-old female patient, with numerous internal diseases in her medical history (symptomatic bradycardia, insulin-dependent diabetes mellitus, atrial fibrillation, history of breast cancer), was admitted to hospital with complaints of sudden vomiting and severe abdominal pain. A prior appendectomy was documented. Clinical symptoms included mildly bloated abdomen and pressure pain in the lower right and left abdomen. No development of peritonitis so far. On an ultrasound scan, massive meteorism could be seen, but presence of free fluid could not be verified. No air-fluid levels could be seen on abdominal X-ray images. Additionally, distinctive aortic calcification. A CT scan showed perihepatic ascites, but no further major pathologies were found. Laboratory tests confirmed marked leukocytosis but only minor elevation of the CRP value. Only now, the lactic acid value was determined and found to be 20 times the norm. The next day, the patient was transferred to a university clinic and

underwent immediate laparotomy, which verified ischemia of the right hemicolon and of the terminal ileum, in conjunction with blackish necrotized stretches of bowel. Discontinuity resection of the right hemicolon was performed, with creation of a terminal ileostomy. Histological tests confirmed extensive ischemic mucosal ulcerations and transmigration peritonitis. The patient died in ICU, due to sepsis-induced multiple organ failure.

Conclusion: Mesenteric ischemia was diagnosed belatedly, after approximately 24 hours. This considerable delay may be considered a culpable error. In this case, based on the patient's condition and diagnostic findings, mesenteric ischemia should have been suspected at a much earlier time.

2.8.10 Summary

The forensic aspects of the treatment of acute abdomen pertain almost exclusively to issues arising from (lack of) result-oriented primary diagnostics, thorough observation of the patient's further clinical progression and timely or belated, indication for surgery. Adequate documentation of clinical findings and transparent decision-making plays a decisive role in juridical evaluations.

References

[1] Clavien, PA, Sanabria, JR, Mentha, G. et al. Recent results of elective open cholecystectomy in a North American and a European Center. Comparison of complications and risk factors. Ann Surg 1992; 216:618–626.
[2] Mühe, E. Long-term follows up after laparoscopic cholecystectomy. Endoscopy 1992; 24: 754–758.
[3] Mühe, E. [Laparoscopic cholecystectomy – late results]. Klin Chir. 1991: 10–13.
[4] Mühe, E. [Laparoscopic cholecystectomy – late results]. Langenbecks Arch Chir Suppl Kongressbd. 1991:416–423.
[5] Mouret, P. How I developed laparoscopic cholecystectomy. Ann Acad Med Singapore. 1996; 25:744–747.
[6] Cuschieri, A, Dubois, F, Mouret, P. et al. The European experience with laparoscopic cholecystectomy. Am J Surg 1991; 161:385–387.
[7] Dubois, F, Berthelot, G, Levard, H. [Laparoscopic cholecystectomy. Technique and complications. Report of 2,665 cases]. Bull Acad Natl Med. 1995; 179:1059–1066; discussion 1066–1068.
[8] Perissat, J, Collet, D, Belliard, R. Gallstones. Laparoscopic treatment – cholecystectomy, cholecystostomy, and lithotripsy. Our own technique. Surg Endosc. 1990; 4:1–5.
[9] NIH Consensus Conference. Gallstones and laparoscopic cholecystectomy. JAMA 1993; 269:1018–1024.
[10] Carey. LC Cholecystectomy – a new standard. Ann Surg 1992; 216:617.
[11] Hardy, KJ. Gallstones and laparoscopic cholecystectomy: a consensus? Aust NZJ Surg. 1994; 64:583–587.
[12] Nakeeb, A, Comuzzie, AG, Martin, L. et al. Gallstones. Genetics versus environment. Ann Surg. 2002; 235:842–849.
[13] Hospital Episode Statistics 2005–2006, May, 2009.
[14] Scurr, JRH, Brigstocke, JR, Shields, DA. et al. Medico legal claims following laparoscopic cholecystectomy in the UK and Ireland. Ann R Coll Surg Engl. 2010; 92:286–291.

[15] Christof-Veit, JB, Döbler, K, Fischer, B. Qualität sichtbar machen. BQS-Qualitätsreport 2008. In: BQS Bundesgeschäftsstelle Qualitätssicherung GmbH, Düsseldorf, 2009; p. 52.

[16] Velanovic, V, Morton, JM, McDonald, M. Analysis of the SAGES outcomes initiative cholecystectomy, registry. Surg Endosc 2006; 20:43–50.

[17] Strasberg, SM, Hertl, M, Soper, NJ. Analysis of the problem of biliary injury during laparoscopic cholecystectomy. J Am Coll Surg. 1995; 180:101–125.

[18] Lau, WY, Lai, ECH. Classification of iatrogenic bile duct injury. Hepatobiliary Pancreat Dis Int, Vol 6, N 5, October 15, 2007.

[19] Flum, D. R., Cheadle, A., Prela, C., Dellinger, E. P., Chan, L. Bile duct injury during cholecystectomy and survival in medicare beneficiaries. JAMA 2003; 290:2168–2173.

[20] Lai, EC, Lau, WY. Mirizzi syndrome: history, present and future development. ANZ J Surg 2006; 76:251–257.

[21] Melton, GB, Lillemoe, KD, Cameron, JL. et al. Major bile duct injuries associated with laparoscopic cholecystectomy: effect of surgical repair on the quality of life. Ann Surg 2002; 235:888–895.

[22] Russell, JC, Walsh, SJ, Mattie, AS, Lynch, JT. Bile duct injuries, 1989–1993. A state-wide experience. Connecticut laparoscopic cholecystectomy registry. Arch Surg. 1996; 131:382–388.

[23] Walsh, RM, Henderson, JM, Vogt, DP, Mayes, JT, Grundfest-Broniatowski, S. et al. Trends in bile duct injuries from laparoscopic cholecystectomy. J Gastrointest Surg. 1998; 2:458–462.

[24] Dolan, JP, Diggs, BS, Sheppard, BG, Hunter, JG. Ten-year trend in the national volume of bile duct injuries requiring operative repair. Surg Endosc. 2005; 19:967–973.

[25] Keus, F, de Jong, JA, Gooszen, HG, van Laarhoven, CJ. Laparoscopic versus open cholecystectomy for patients with symptomatic cholecystolithiasis. Cochrane Database Syst Rev 2006; CD006231.

[26] Kang, JY, Ellis, C, Majeed, A. et al. Gallstone – an increasing problem: a study of hospital admissions in England between 1989/1990 and 1999/2000. Aliment Pharmacol Ther. 2003; 17:561–569.

[27] Hüttl, TP, Hrdina, C, Geiger, TK, Meyer, G, Schildberg, FW. et al. Management of Common bile duct stones – Results of a nationwide survey with analysis of 8433 common bile duct explorations in Germany. Zentralblatt für Chirurgie 2002; 127:282–288.

[28] Livingstone, EH, Rege, RV. Technical Complications are arising as common duct exploration is becoming rare. Journal of the American College of Surgeons, 2005; 201:426–433.

[29] Roslyn, JJ, Binns, GS, Hughes, EF. et al. Open cholecystectomy: a contemporary analysis of 42,474 patients. Ann Surg. 1993; 218:129–137.

[30] Deziel, DJ, Millikan, KW, Economou, SG. et al. Complications of laparoscopic cholecystectomy: a national survey of 4,292 hospitals and an analysis of 77,604 cases. Am J Surg. 1993; 165:9–14.

[31] Wherry, DC, Marohn, MR, Malanoski, MP. et al. An external audit of laparoscopic cholecystectomy in the steady state performed in medical treatment facilities of the Department of Defense. Ann Surg. 1996; 224:145–154.

[32] Orlando, R, 3rd, Russel, JC, Lynch, J. et al. Laparoscopic cholecystectomy: a state-wide experience: the Connecticut Laparoscopic Cholecystectomy Registry. Arch Surg. 1993; 128: 494–498.

[33] Wherry, DC, Rob, CG, Marohn, MR. et al. An external audit of laparoscopic cholecystectomy performed in medical treatment facilities of the Department of Defense. Ann Surg. 1994; 220:626–634.

[34] Go, PM, Schol, F, Gouma, DJ. Laparoscopic cholecystectomy in the Netherlands. Br J Surg. 1993; 80:1180–1183.

[35] Lillemoe, KD, Melton, GB, Cameron, JL. et al. Postoperative bile duct strictures: management and outcome in the 1990s. Ann Surg. 2000; 232:430–441.

[36] Calvete, J, Sabater, L, Camps, B. et al: Bile duct injury during laparoscopic cholecystectomy: myth or reality of the learning curve? Surg Endosc. 2000; 14:608–611.

[37] Sicklich, JK, Camps, MS, Lillemoe, KD, Melton, GB. et al. Surgical management of bile duct injuries sustained during laparoscopic cholecystectomy. Ann Surg. 2005; Vol 241, No 5.

[38] Böhm, B, Schwenk, W, Junghans, T. Das Pneumoperitoneum, Auswirkungen der Laparoskopie auf die Organsysteme. 2000; Springer-Verlag.

[39] Schäfer, M, Lauper, M, Krähenbühl, L. Trocar and verres needle injuries during laparoscopic. Surg Endosc 2001; 15:275.

[40] Orlando, R, Palatini, P, Lirussi, F. Needle and trokar injuries in diagnostic laparoscopy under local anaesthesia: what is the true incidence of these complications? Laparoendosc Adv Surg Tech 2003; A 13:181.

[41] Sigman, HH, Fried, GM, Garzon, J. et al. Risks of blind versus open approach to celiotomy for laparoscopic surgery. Surg Laparos Endosc 1993; 3:296.

[42] Ballem, RV, Rudomanski, J. Techniques of Pneumoperitoneum. Surg Laparosc Endosc 1993; 3:42.

[43] Adamsen, S, Hansen, OH, Funch-Jensen, P. et al. Bile duct injury during laparoscopic cholecystectomy. a prospective nationwide series. J Am Coll Surg 1997; 184:571.

[44] Helme, S, Samdani, T, Sinha, P. Complications of spilled gallstones following laparoscopic cholecystectomy: a case report and literature overview. J Med Case Reports 2009; 3:8626.

[45] Bhatti, CS, Tamijmarane, A, Bramhall, SR. A tale of three spilled gallstones: one liver mass and two abscesses. Dig Surg 2006; 23:198–200.

[46] Chandler, JG, Voyles, CR, Floore, TH. et al. Litigious consequences of open and laparoscopic biliary surgical mishaps. J Gastrointest Surg. 1997; 1:138–145.

[47] Pankaj, GR, Soonawalla, ZF, Grant, HW. Medico legal costs of bile duct injuries incurred during laparoscopic cholecystectomy. HPB (Oxford). 2009; March; 11 (2):130–134.

[48] Bismuth, H, Lazorthes, F. Les traumatismes opératoires de la voie biliaire principale. 1982; Masson, Paris.

[49] Bergman, JJ, van den Brink, GR, Rauws, EA, de Wit, L, Obertop, H, Huibregtse, K. et al. Treatment of bile duct lesions after laparoscopic cholecystectomy. Gut 1996; 38:141–147.

[50] Neuhaus, P, Schmidt, SC, Hintze, RE, Adler, A, Veltzke, W, Raakow, R. et al. Classification and treatment of bile duct injuries after laparoscopic cholecystectomy. Chirurg 2000; 71:166–173.

[51] Csendes, A, Navarrete, C, Burdiles, P, Yarmuch, J. Treatment of common bile duct injuries during laparoscopic cholecystectomy: endoscopic and surgical management. World J Surg 2001; 25:1346–1351.

[52] Stewart, L, Robinson, TN, Lee, CM, Liu, K, Whang, K, Way, LW. Right hepatic artery injury associated with laparoscopic bile duct injury: incidence, mechanism, and consequences. J Gastrointest Surg 2004; 8:523–531.

[53] Catarci, M, Carlini, M, Gentileschi, P. et al. Major and minor injuries during the creation of Pneumoperitoneum. A multicenter study on 12,919 cases. Surg Endosc. 2001; 15:566–569.

[54] Jansen, FW, Kolkman, W, Bakkum, EA. et al. Complications of laparoscopy: an inquiry about closed – versus open – entry technique. Am J Obstet Gynecol 2004; 190:634–638.

[55] Strasberg, SM. Error traps and vasculobiliary injury in laparoscopic and open cholecystectomy. J Hepatobiliary Pancreat Surg 2008; 15:284–292.

[56] Way, S, Stewart, L, Gantert, W. et al. Causes and prevention of laparoscopic bile duct injuries: analysis of 252 cases from a human factors and cognitive psychology perspective. Ann Surg 2003; 237:460–469.

[57] Strasberg, SM, Brunt, LM. Rationale and use of the critical view of safety in laparoscopic cholecystectomy. J Am Coll Surg 2010; 211:132–138.

[58] Davidoff, AM, Pappas, TN, Murray, EA. et al. Mechanism of major biliary injury during laparoscopic cholecystectomy. Am J Surg. 1992; 215:196–298.

[59] Al-Kubati, WR. Bile duct injury following laparoscopic cholecystectomy. A Clinical Study Saudi J Gastroenterol. 2010 April; 16 (2), 100–104.

[60] Goldstein, EB. Sensation and perception, 6th ed. Pacific grove, CA: Wadsworth 2002.

[61] Madariaga, JR, Dodson, SF, Selby, R, Todo, S. et al. Corrective treatment and anatomic considerations for laparoscopic cholecystectomy injuries. J Am Coll Surg: 1994 September; 179(3):321–325.

[62] Neuhaus, P, Schmidt, SC, Hintze, RE, Adler, A, Bechstein, WO. Einteilung und Behandlung von Gallengangsverletzungen nach laparoskopischer Cholezystektomie. Chirurg 2000; 71: 166–173.

[63] Blumgart, LH, Kelley, CJ, Benjamin, IS. Benign bile duct stricture following cholecystectomy: critical factors in management. Br J Surg 1984; 71:836.

[64] Chapman, WC, Halevy, A, Blumgart, LH, Benjamin, IS. Postcholecystectomy bile duct strictures. Arch Surg 1995; 130:597.

[65] Hellinger, A, Lange, R, Peitgen, K, Stephan, V. et al. Gallengangsläsionen bei laparoskopischer Cholezystektomie – Rekonstruktionsverfahren und Ergebnisse. Zentralbl Chir 1997; 122:1092.

[66] Pellegrini, CA, Thomas, MJ, Way, LW. Recurrent biliary stricture. Patterns of recurrence and outcome of surgical therapy. Am J Surg 1983; 147:175.

[67] Raute, M, Podlech, P, Jaschke, W, Manegold, BC. et al. Management of bile duct injury and strictures following cholecystectomy. World J Surg 1993; 17:553.

[68] Davids, PHP, Ringers, J, Rauws, EAJ, de Wit, LT. et al. Bile duct inury after laparoscopic cholecystectomy the value of endoscopic retrograde cholangiopancreaticography. Gut 1993; 34:1250.

[69] Gigot, JF, Etienne, J, Aerts, R, Wibin, E. et al. The dramatic reality of biliary tract injury during laparoscopic cholecystectomy. An anonymous multicenter Belgian survey of 65 patients. Surg Endosc 1997; 11:1171.

[70] Berner. Anzahl von Begutachtungen im Rahmen der Behandlung eines Gallensteinleidens. Personal Communication, German Medical Association 2009; Berlin.

[71] Francoeur, JR, Wiseman, K, Buczkowski, AK. et al. Surgeons' anonymous response after bile duct injury during cholecystectomy. Am J Surg 2003; 185:468–475.

[72] Massarweh, NN, Flum, DR. Role of intraoperative cholangiography in avoiding bile duct injury. J Am Coll Surg 2007; 204:656–664.

[73] Fellmer, PT, Fellmer, J, Jonas, S. Arzthaftung bei Gallengangsverletzungen nach laparoskopischer Cholezystektomie. Chirurg 2011; 82:68–73.

[74] McLean, TR. Risk management observations from litigation involving laparoscopic cholecystectomy. Arch Surg 2006; 141:643–648.

[75] Kern, KA. Malpractice litigation involving laparoscopic cholecystectomy. Cost, cause, and consequences. Arch Surg 1997; 132:392–397. Discussion 397–398.

[76] Physician Insurers Association of America. Rockville, M.D.: Physician Insurers Association of America Laparoscopic Procedure Study.

[77] Roy, PG, Soonawalla, ZF, Grant, H. Medico legal costs of bile duct injuries incurred during laparoscopic cholecystectomy. HPB (Oxford), 2009 March; 11(2):130–134.

[78] Kern, KA. Medico-legal analysis of bile duct injury during open cholecystectomy and abdominal surgery. Am J Surg. 1994; 168:217–222.

[79] Carroll, BJ, Birth, M, Phillips, EH. Common bile duct injuries during laparoscopic cholecystectomy that result in litigation. Surg Endosc. 1998; 12:310–313. Discussion 314.

[80] Ferriman, A. Laparoscopic surgery: two thirds of injuries initially missed. BMJ 2000; 321(7264):784.

[81] Büter, F. Inauguraldissertation „Sogenannte Kunstfehler" im Sektionsgut des Institutes für Rechtsmedizin in Hamburg (2002–2006) unter besonderer Berücksichtigung endoskopischer und laparoskopischer Eingriffe. Hamburg 2009.

[82] De Reuver, PR, Dijkgraat, MG, Gevers, SK. et al. Poor agreement among expert witnesses in bile duct injury malpractice litigation: an expert panel survey. Ann Surg 2008; 248:815–820.

[83] Ruling of the Higher District Court (OLG) Hamm from 28.11.2008, file reference 26 and 28/08. In: GesR 2009:247–248.

[84] Lillemoe, KD. To err is human, but should we expect more from a surgeon? Ann Surg 2003; 237:470–471.

[85] Fischer, JE. Is damage to the common bile duct during laparoscopic cholecystectomy an inherent risk of the operation? Am J Surg 2009; 197:829–832.

[86] May, T, Aulisio, MP. Medical malpractice mistake prevention, and compensation. Kennedy Inst. Ethics J. 2001; 11:134–146.

[87] DeVita, MA, Aulisio, MP. The ethics of medical mistakes: historical, legal, and institutional perspectives. Kennedy Inst. Ethics J. 2001; 11:115–116.

[88] Perrow, C. Normal accidents. Living with high-risk technologies. Princeton, N.J., Princeton University Press, 1999.

[89] Fletscher, DR, Hobbs, MS, Tan, P. et al. Complications of cholecystectomy: risks of the laparoscopic approach and protective effects of operative cholangiography: a population-based study. Ann Surg. 1999; 229:449–457.

[90] Woods, MS, Traverso, LW, Kozarek, RA. et al. Biliary tract complications of laparoscopic cholecystectomy are detected more frequently with routine intraoperative cholangiography. Surg Endosc. 1995; 110:1076–1080.

[91] Connor, S, Garden, OJ. Bile duct injury in the era of laparoscopic cholecystectomy. Br J Surg. 2006; 93:158–68.

[92] Dekker, SW, Hugh, TB. Laparoscopic bile duct injury: understanding the psychology and heuristics of the error. ANZ J Surg 2008; 78:1109–1114.

[93] Strasberg, SM. Biliary injury in laparoscopic surgery: part 1. Processes used in determination of standard of care in misidentification injuries. J Am Coll Surg. 2005; 201:598–603.

[94] Strasberg, SM. Biliary injury in laparoscopic surgery: part 2. Changing the culture of cholecystectomy. J Am Coll Surg. 2005; 201:604–611.

[95] Ruling of the Higher Disrict Court (OLG) Schleswig-Holstein from 29.05.2009, file reference 4 V 38108. In: OLG Schleswig 2009:594–597.

[96] Bauch, J, Bruch, HP, Heberer, J, Jähne, J. Behandlungsfehler und Haftpflicht in der Viszeralchirurgie. Springer Verlag Heideberg, 2011.

[97] Sturm, J, Post, S. Benigne Erkrankungen der Gallenblase und Gallenwege. Chirurg 2000; 71:1530–1551.

[98] Mussack, T, Trupka, AW, Schmidbauer, S, Hallfeldt, KKJ. Zeitgerechtes Management von Gallengangkomplikationen nach laparoskopischer Cholezystektomie. Chirurg 2000; 71:174–181.

[99] Schmidt, SC, Langrehr, JM, Hintze, RE, Neuhaus, P. Long term results and risk factors influencing outcome of major bile duct injuries following cholecystectomy. Br J Surg 2005; 93:76–82.

[100] Hand, AA, Self, ML, Dunn, E. Abdominal wall abscess formation two years after laparoscopic cholecystectomy. Jour Adv Lap Surg 2006; 10:105–107.

[101] Conciliation Committee of the State Chamber of Medicine in Rhineland-Palatinate. Proceedings 003/07. Published 02.05.2008. "Ärzteblatt Rhineland-Pfalz", January 2011, Vol. 1, p. 17.

[102] Vinz, H. Communication from the Conciliation Body of the Northern German State Chamber of Medicine. Schleswig-Holsteinisches Ärzteblatt 2002; 06.

[103] Catarci, M, Carlini, M, Gentileschi, P. et al. Major and minor injuries during the creation of pneumoperitoneum. A multicenter Study on 12,919 cases. Surg Endosc 2001; 15:566–569.

[104] Hallfeldt, KKJ, Schmidbauer, S, Trupka, A. Optical trocars types, indications, clinical experiences. Min Invas Ther Allied Technol 2001; 10:47–50.

[105] Hasson, HM, Rotman, C, Rana, N, Kumari, NA. Open laparoscopy: 29-year-experience. Obstet Gynecol 2000; 96:763–766.

[106] Jirecek, S, Drager, M, Leitich, H. et al. Direct visual or blind insertion of the primary trocar. Surg Endosc. 2002; 16:626–629.

[107] Schmedt, CG, Leibl, BJ, Däubler, P, Bittner, R. Access-related complications – analysis of 6,023 consecutive laparoscopic hernia repairs. Min invas. The Allied Technol 2001; 10: 23–30.

[108] String, A, Berber, E, Foroutani, A. et al. Use of the optical access trocar for safe and rapid entry in various laparoscopic procedures. Surg Endosc. 2001; 15:570–573.

[109] Dunn, DC, Watson, CJE. Disposable guarded trocar and cannular in laparoscopic surgery: a caveat. Br J Surg. 1992; 79:927.

[110] Bonjer, HJ, Hazebroek, EJ, Kazemier, G. et al. Open versus closed establishment of Pneumo-peritoneum in laparoscopic surgery. Br J Surg. 1997; 84:599.

[111] Esposito, C. Influence of different trocar tips on abdominal wall penetration during laparo-scopy. Surg Endosc. 1998; 12:1434.

[112] Hallfeldt, K, Trupka, A, Kalteis, T. et al. Laparoscopic needles and trocars: an overview of designs and complications. J Laparoendosc. Surg. 1992; 2-117–125.

[113] Hashizume, M, Sugimachi, K. Needle and trocar injury during laparoscopic surgery in Japan. Surg. Endosc. 1997; 11:1198.

[114] Schaller, G, Kuenkel, M, Manegold, BC. Serious trocar accidents in laparoscopic surgery: a French survey of 103,852 operations. Surg Laparosc Endosc 1996; 6:367.

[115] Bhoyrul, S, Payne J, Steffens, B. et al. A randomized prospective study of radially expanding trocars in laparoscopic surgery. J Gastrointest Surg 2000; 4:302–397.

[116] Chaprou, C, Pierre, F, Querleu, D. et al. Major vascular complications from gynaecologic laparoscopy. Gynecol Obstet Fertil 2000; 28:880–887.

[117] Germer, CT, Ritz, JP, Buhr, HJ. Laparoskopische Kolonchirurgie. Chirurg 2003; 74:966–982.

[118] Wichmann, MW, Meyer, G, Angele, MK. et al. Recent advances in minimally invasive colorectal cancer surgery. Onkologe 2002; 25:318–323.

[119] Hohenberger, W, Merkel, S. Die laparoskopische Chirurgie des Kolonkarzinoms. Chirurg 2004; 75:1052–1055.

[120] Nelson, H, Sargent, DJ, Wieland, S. et al. A comparison of laparoscopically assisted and open colectomy for colon cancer. N Engl J Med 2004; 350:2050–2059.

[121] Weeks, JC, Nelson, H, Gelber, S. et al. Short-term quality-of-life-outcomes following laparo-scopic assisted colectomy vs open colectomy for colon cancer. A randomized trial. JAMA 2002; 287:321–328.

[122] Janson, M, Björholt, I, Carlsson, P. et al. Randomized Clinical trial of the costs of open and laparoscopic surgery for colonic cancer. Br J Surg 2004; 91:409–417.

[123] Franklin, ME, Rosenthal, D, Abrego-Medina et al. Prospective comparison of open vs lap-aroscopic colon surgery for carcinoma. Five-year results. Dis Colon Rectum 1996; 39: 10 [Suppl]:35–46.

[124] Fusco, MA, Paluzzi, MW. Abdominal wall recurrence after laparoscopic assisted colec-tomy for de-novo carcinom of the colon. Report of a case. Dis Colon Rektum 1993; 36: 858–861.

[125] Wexner, SD, Cohen, SM. Port site metastases after laparoscopic colorectal surgery for cure of malignancy. Br J Surg 1995; 82:295–8.

[126] Lacy, AM, Delgado, S, García-Valdecasa, JC. et al. Port-site metasases and recurrence after laparoscopic colectomy. A randomized trial. Surg Endosc 1998 Aug; 12 (8): 1039–42.

[127] Milsom, JW, Böhm, B, Hammerhofer, KA, Fazio V. et al. A prospective vs conventional techniques in colorectal cancer surgery: a preliminary report. JAMA Coll Surg 1998; 187: 55–7.

[128] Montz, FJ, Holschneider, CH, Munro, MG. Incisional hernia following laparoscopy: a survey of the American association of gynaecologic laparoscopists. Obstet Gynecol 1994; 84:881.

[129] Ridings, P, Evans, DS. The transabdominal pre-peritoneal (TAPP) inguinal hernia repair: a trip along the learning curve. IR Coll Surg Edingb 2000; 45:29.

[130] Holzinger, F, Klaiber, C. Trokarhernien. Chirurg 2002; 73:899–904.

[131] Leibl, BJ, Schmedt, CG, Schwarz, J, Kraft, K. et al. Laparoscopic surgery complications associated with trocar tip design: review of literature and own results. J Laparoendosc Adv Surg Tech-Part A, 1999; vol. 9, no. 2, pp.135–140.

[132] Krug, F, Herold, A, Wenk, H, Bruch, HP. Narbenhernien nach laparoskopischen Eingriffen. Chirurg 1995; 66:419.

[133] Plaus, WJ. Laparoscopic trocar site hernias. J Laparoendosc Surg 1993; 3:567.

[134] Boike, GM, Miller, CE, Spirtos, NM. et al. Incisional bowel herniations after operative laparoscopy: a series of nineteen cases and review of the literature. Am J Obstet Gynecol 1995; 6:1726.

[135] Lajer, H, Widecrantz, S, Heisterberg, L. Hernias in trocar ports following abdominal laparoscopy. Acta Obstet Gynecol Scand 1997; 76:389.

[136] Rastogi, V, Dy, V. Simple technique for proper approximation and closure of peritoneal and rectus sheat defects at port site after laparoscopic surgery. J Laparoendosc Adv Surg Techn 2001; A 11:13.

[137] Bhoyrul, S, Payne, J, Steffens, B, Swanstrom, L, Way, LW. A randomized prospective study of radially expanding trocars in laparoscopic surgery. J Gastrointest Surg 4:392.

[138] Kolmorgen, K. Prävention von Laparoskopie-Komplikationen aus gutachterlicher Sicht: Gynäkologie 2002; 35:495–500.

[139] Schein, M, Wittmann, DH, Aprahamian, CC. et al. The abdominal compartment syndrome: the physiological and clinical consequences of elevated intraabdominal pressure. J Am Surg 1995; 180:745–753.

[140] Caldwell, CB, Ricotta, JJ. Changes in visceral blood flow with elevated intraabdominal pressure. J Surg Res 1987; 43:14–20.

[141] Wassenaar, EB, Raymakers, JT, Rakia, S. Fatal intestinal ischemia after laparoscopic correction of incisional hernia. JSLS 2007; Jul-Sept; 11(3):389–393.

[142] Hoffmann, J, Jauch, KW. Chirurgie der Appendizitis. In: Bauch, J, Bruch, HP, Heberer, J, Jähne, J (ed). Behandlungsfehler und Haftpflicht in der Viszeralchirurgie. Springer-Verlag 2011; 278–279.

[143] Rutkow, J. M. Epidemiologic, economic and sociologic aspects of hernia surgery in the United States in the 1990s. Surg Clin North Am 1998; 78:941–951.

[144] Nyhus, LM, Condon, RE. Hernia 4th ed. Lippincott Philadelphia 1995.

[145] Miserez, M, Alexandre, JH, Campanelli, G. et al. The European hernia society groin hernia classification: Simple and easy to remember. Hernia. 2007; 11:113–116.

[146] Bassini, E. Über die Behandlung des Leistenbruches. Arch Klin Chir 1890; 40:429.

[147] Amid, PK, Shulman, AG, Lichtenstein, EL. Die Herniotomie nach Lichtenstein. Chirurg 1994; 65:54.

[148] Lichtenstein, EL, Shore, JM. Simplified repair of femoral and recurrent inguinal hernias by a „plug-technic". Am J Surg 1974; 128:439.

[149] Glassow, F. Short-stay surgery for repair of inguinal hernia. Ann R Coll Surg Engl 1976; 58:133.

[150] Stoppa, RE, Rives, JL, Warlaumont, CR. et al. The use of Dacron in the repair of hernias of the groin surgery. Clin North Am 1984; 64:269.

[151] Amid, PK, Shulman, AG, Lichtenstein, IL. Critical scrutiny of the open tension-free hernioplasty. Am J Surg 1993; 165:369.

[152] Stoppa, RE, Warlaumont, CR. The peritoneal approach and prosthetic repair of the groin hernia. In: Nyhus, LM, Condon, RE. (eds) Hernia, 3rd ed. Lippincott, Philadelphia 1989; p 199.

[153] Bauch, J, Bruch, HP, Jähne, J (ed). Behandlungsfehler und Haftpflicht in der Viszeralchirurgie. Springer 2011.

[154] Jähne, J. Chirurgie der Leistenhernie. Chirurg 2001; 72:456–471.

[155] Hansis, ML. Begutachtung vorgeworfener Behandlungsfehler – „das gute Gutachten". MED SACH 2006; 102:10–15.

[156] Lichtenstein, IL, Shulman, AG, Amid, PK. et al. Cause and prevention of postherniorrhaphy neuralgia: a proposed protocol for treatment. Am J Surg 1988; 155:786–90.

[157] Heise, CP, Starling, JR. Mesh inguinodynia: a new clinical syndrome after inguinal herniorraphy? J Am Surg 1998; 187:514–8.

[158] Bower, S, Moore, BB, Weiss, SM. Neuralgia after inguinal hernia repair. Am Surg 1996; 62: 664–7.

[159] Liem, MS, van der Graaf, Y, van Steensel, CJ. et al. Comparison of conventional anterior surgery and laparoscopic surgery for inguinalhernia repair. N Engl J Med 1997; 336: 1541–7.

[160] Grant, AM, Scott, NW, O'Dywer, PJ. On behalf of the MRC Laparoscopic Groin Hernia Trial Group Five-year follow-up of a randomized trial to asses pain and numbness after laparoscopic or open repair of groin hernia. Br J of Surg 2004; 91:1570–4.

[161] Wright, D, Paterson, C, Scott, N, Hair, A, O'Dywer, PJ. Five-Year Follow-Up of Patients Undergoing Laparoscopic or Open Groin Hernia Repair. A Randomized Controlled Trial. Ann of Surg 2002; 235:333–7.

[162] McCormack, K, Scott, NW, Go, PM, Ross, S. et al. The EU Trialists Collaboration laparoscopic techniques versus open techniques for inguinal hernia repair. Cochrane Database. Syst Rev. 2003: CD001785.

[163] Fitzgibbons, RJ, Jr, Camps, J, Cornet, DA. et al. Laparoscopic inguinal herniorrhaphy. Results of a multicenter trial. Ann Surg 1995, January; 221(1):3–13.

[164] Scott, NW, McCormack, K, Graham, P. Open mesh versus non-mesh for repair of femoral and inguinal hernia. Chochrane Database Syst Rev 2002; CD002197.

[165] The EU Hernia Trialists Collaboration. Repair of groin hernia with synthetic mesh: Meta-analysis of randomized controlled trials. Ann Surg 2002; 235:322–332.

[166] Lauscher, JC, Yafaei, K, Buhr, HJ. et al. Totale extraperitoneale Hernioplastik. Chirurg 2009; 80:956–965.

[167] Fränneby, U, Sandblom, G, Nordin, P. et al. Risk factors for long-term pain after hernia surgery. Ann Surg. 2006; 244:212–219.

[168] Massaron, S, Bona, S, Fumaqalli U. et al. Long-term sequelae after 1,311 primary inguinal hernia repairs. Hernia 2008; 12:57–63.

[169] Kalliomäki, ML, Meyerson, J, Gunnarsson, U. et al. Long-term pain after inguinal hernia repair in a population-based cohort; risk factors and interference with daily activities. Eur J Pain 2008; 12:214–225.

[170] Loos, MJ, Roumen, RM, Scheltinga, MR. Chronic sequelae of common elective groin hernia repair. Hernia 2007; 11:169–173.

[171] Callesen, T, Bech, K, Kehlet, H. Prospective study of chronic pain after groin hernia repair. Br J Surg 1999; 86:1528–1531.

[172] Poobalan, AS, Bruce, J, King, PM. et al. Chronic pain and quality of life following open inguinal hernia repair. Br J Surg 2001; 88:1122–1126.

[173] Page, B, Paterson, C, Young, D, O'Dywer, PJ. Pain from primary inguinal hernia and the effect of repair on pain. Br J Surg 2002; 89:1315–1318.

[174] Grant, AM, Scott, NW, O'Dywer, PJ. MRC Laparoscopic Groin Hernia Trial Group. Five-year-follow-up of a randomized trial to assess pain and numbness after laparoscopic or open repair of groin hernia. Br J Surg 2004; 91:1570–1574.

[175] van Veen, RN, Wijsmuller, AR, Vrijland, WW. et al. Randomized clinical trial of mesh versus non-mesh primary inguinal hernia repair: Long-term chronic pain at 10 years. Surgery 2007; 142:695–698.

[176] Lauscher, JC, Buhr, HJ, Gröne, J. Erfahrungen aus über 2,100 Hernienreparationen. Chirurg 2011; 82:255–262.

[177] Lammers, BJ, Meyer, HJ, Huber, HG. Entwicklungen bei der Leistenhernie vor dem Hintergrund neu eingeführter Eingriffstechniken im Kammerbereich. Nordrhein Chirurg 2001; 72:441–452.

[178] Schumpelick, V. Leistenbruchreparation nach Shouldice 1984; Chirurg 55:25–28.

[179] Felix, EL, Michas, CA, Gonzalez, MH. Laparoscopic hernioplasty; TAPP vs TEP. Surg Endosc 1995; 9:984.

[180] Felix, EL, Michas, CA, McKnight, RK. Laparoscopic herniorrhaphy; transabdominal preperitoneal floor repair. Surg Endosc 1994; 8:100.

[181] Vader, VL, Vogt, DM, Zucker, KA, Thilstead, JP, Curet, MJ. Adhesion formation in laparoscopic inguinal hernia repair. Surg Endosc 1997; 11:825.

[182] Bittner, R, Kraft, K, Schwarz, J, Leibl, B. Risiko und Nutzen der Laparoskopischen Hernioplastik (TAPP), 5 Jahre Erfahrungen bei 3,400 Hernienreparationen. Chirurg 1998; 69:854.

[183] Chiofalo, R, Holzinger, F, Klaiber, C. Total extraperitoneale Netzplastik bei primären und Rezidivhernien – Gibt es Unterschiede? Chirurg 2001; 72:1485.

[184] Gerber, S, Hämmerli, PA, Glättli, A. Laparoskopische transabdominale präperitoneale Hernioplastik-Evaluation der zugangsbedingten Komplikationen. Chirurg 2000; 71:824.

[185] Kapiris, SA, Brough, WA, Royston, CMS, O'Boyle, C, Sedman, PC. Laparoscopic transperitoneal (TAPP) hernia repair – a 7-year two-center experience in 3,017 patients. Surg Endosc 2001; 15:972.

[186] Schultz, C, Baca, I, Götzen, V. Laparoscopic inguinal hernia repair – a review of 2,500 cases. Surg Endosc 2001; 15:582.

[187] Stoppa, RE, Warlaumont, CR. The preperitoneal approach and prosthetic repair of the groin hernia. In: Nyhus, L. M., Condon, R. E. (eds) Hernia 1989; 3rd ed. Lippincott, Philadelphia, p 199.

[188] Fitzgibbons, RJ, Camps, J, Cornet, DA, Nguyen, NX. et al. Laparoscopic Inguinal Herniorrhaphy – results of a multicenter trial. Ann Surg 1995; 221:3.

[189] Klaiber, C, Banz, M, Metzger, A. Die Technik der endoskopischen präperitonealen Netzplastik zur Behandlung der Hernien der Leistenregion (TEP). Minim Invasive Chir 1999; 8:86.

[190] Schumpelick, V, Töns, C, Kupcyk-Joeris, D. Operation der Leistenhernie, Klassifikation, Verfahrenswahl, Technik und Ergebnisse. Chirurg 1991; 62:641.

[191] Felix, EL, Scott, S, Crafton, B, Geis, P. et al. Causes of recurrence after laparoscopic hernioplasty. A multicenter study. Surg Endosc 1998; 12:226.

[192] Tan, GH, Gharib, H. Thyroid incidentalomas: management approaches to non-palpable nodules discovered incidentally on thyroid imaging. Ann Intern Med 1997; 126:226–231.

[193] Enderlen, E, Hotz, G. Beiträge zur Anatomie der Struma und zur Kropfoperation. Z Angew Anat 1918; 3:57–79.

[194] Dralle, H. Rekurrens- und Nebenschilddrüsenpräparation in der Schilddrüsenchirurgie. Chirurg 2009; 80:352–363.

[195] Delbridge, L, Guinea, AL, Reeve, TS. Total thyroidectomy for bilateral benign multinodular goiter: effect of changing practice. Arch Surg 1999; 134:1389–1393.

[196] Liu, Q, Djuricin, G, Prinz. RA. Total thyroidectomy for benign thyroid disease. Surgery 1998; 123:2–7.

[197] Reeve, TS, Delbridge, L, Lohen, A. et al. Total thyroidectomy: the preferred option for multinodular goiter. Ann Surg 1987; 206:782–786.

[198] Thomusch, Q, Sekulla, C, Dralle, H. Rolle der totalen Thyreoidektomie im primären Therapiekonzept der benignen Knotenstruma. Chirurg 2003; 74:437–442.

[199] Wheeler, MH. Total thyroidectomy for benign thyroid disease. Lancet 1998; 35:1626–1627.

[200] Jacobs, J, Aland, J, Ballinger, J. Total thyroidectomy: a review of 213 patients. Ann Surg 1983; 197:542.

[201] Perzik, SL, Katz, B. The place of total thyroidectomy in the management of thyroid disease. Surgery 1967; 62:436.

[202] Steinmüller, T, Ulrich, R, Rayes, N. et al. Operationsverfahren und Risikofaktoren in der Therapie der benignen Struma multinodosa. Chirurg 2001; 72:1453.

[203] Pappalardo, G, Guadalaxara, A, Frattaroli, FM. et al. Total compared which subtotal thyroidectomy in benign nodular disease: personal series and review of published reports. Eur J Surg 1998; 164:501.

[204] Clark, OH. TSH suppression in the management of thyroid nodules and thyroid cancer. World J Surg 1981; 5:39.

[205] Anderson, PE, Hurley, PR, Rosswick, P. Conservative treatment and long term prophylactic thyroxine in the prevention of recurrence of multinodular goiter. Surg Gynecol Obstet 1990; 171:309.

[206] Geerdsen, JP, Hee, P. Non toxic goitre. A study of the pituitary thyroid axis in 14 recurrent cases. Acta Chir Scand 1982; 148:221.

[207] Dralle, H, Pichlmayr, R. Risikominderung bei Rezidiveingriffen wegen benigner Struma. Chirurg 1991; 62:169.

[208] Dumont, JE, Lamy, F, Roger, P, Maenhaut, C. Physiological and pathological regulation of thyroid cell proliferation and differentiation by thyrotropin and other factors. Physiol. Rev 1992; 72:667.

[209] Feldkamp, J, Seppel, T, Becker, A. et al. Jodide or L-thyroxine to prevent recurrent goiter in an iodine-deficient area: prospective sonographic study. World J Surg 1997; 21:10.

[210] Goretzki, PE, Simon, D, Dotzenrath, C. et al. Growth regulation of thyroid and thyroid tumors in humans. World J Surg 2000; 24:193.

[211] Zambudio, AR, Rodriquez, JR, Riquelme, J. et al. Prospective Study of postoperative Complications after total thyroidectomy for multinodular goiters by surgeons with experience in Endocrine Surgery. Ann Surg 2004 July; 240(1):18–25.

[212] Gardiner, KR, Russell, CF. Thyroidectomy for large multinodular colloid goitre. J R Coll Surg Edinbg. 1995; 40:367–370.

[213] Mishra, A, Agarwal, A, Agarwal, G, Mishra, SK. Total thyroidectomy for benign thyroid disorders in an endemic region. World J Surg 2001; 25:307–310.

[214] Menegaux, F, Turpin, G, Dahman, M. et al. Secondary thyroidectomy in patients with prior thyroid surgery for benign disease: a study of 203 cases. Surgery 1999; 125:479–483.

[215] Sosa, JA, Bowman, HM, Tielsch, JM. et al. The importance of surgeon experience for clinical and economic outcomes from thyroidectomy. Ann Surg 1998; 228:320–330.

[216] Bergamaschi, R, Becouam, G, Ronceray, J, Arnaud, JP. Morbidity of thyroid surgery. Am J Surg 1998; 176:71–75.

[217] Hisham, AN, Azlina, AF, Aina, EN. et al. Total thyroidectomy: the procedure of choice for multinodular goiter. Eur J Surg 2001; 167:403–405.

[218] Bononi, M, de Cesare, A, Atella, F. et al. Surgical treatment of multinodular goiter: incidence of lesions of the recurrent nerves after total thyroidectomy. Int Surg 2000; 85:190–193.

[219] Röher, HD, Horster, FA, Frilling, A. et al. Morphologie und funktionsgerechte Chirurgie verschiedener Hyperthyreoseformen. Chirurg 1991; 62:176.

[220] Akerström, G, Malmaeus, J, Bergstrom, R. Surgical anatomy of human parathyroid glands. Surgery 1984; 95:14.

[221] Kern, KA. Medicolegal analysis of errors in diagnosis and treatment of surgical endocrine disease. Surgery 1993; 114:1167–74.

[222] Kienzle, HF, Weltrich, H. Lähmung der Stimmbandnerven nach Schilddrüsenresektion. Dtsch Ärztebl. 2001; 98:A43–A46.

[223] Schulte, KM, Röher, HD. Behandlungsfehler bei Operationen der Schilddrüse. Chirurg 1999; 70:1131–1138.

[224] Wienke, A, Janke, K. Darstellung des Nervus recurrens bei einer Schilddrüsenoperation. Widerstreit zwischen chirurgischer Schule und HNO-Schule. Ruling by the Higher District Court (OLG) Düsseldorf from 25.01.2007 – I-8 U 115/05. Laryngo-Rhino-Otol 2007; 80:595–596.

[225] Katz, AD, Nemiroff, P. Anastomoses and bifurcations of the recurrent laryngeal nerve – report of 1,177 nerves visualized. Am Surg 1993; 59:188–191.

[226] Kruse, E, Olthoff, A, Schiel, R. Functional anatomy of the recurrent and superior laryngeal nerve. Langenbecks Arch Surg 2006; 391:4–8.

[227] Yalçin, B, Tunali, S, Ozan, H. Extralaryngeal division of the recurrent laryngeal nerve: a new description for the inferior laryngeal nerve. Surg Radiol Anat 2008; 30:215–220.

[228] Yalçin, B, Ozan, H. Relationship between the Zuckerkandl's tubercle and entrance point of the inferior laryngeal nerve. Clin Anat 2007; 20:640–643.

[229] Yalçin, B, Poyrazoglu, Y, Ozan, H. Relationship between the Zuckerkandl's tubercle and the inferior laryngeal nerve including the laryngeal branches. Surg Today 2007; 37: 109–113.

[230] Deutsche Gesellschaft für Chirurgie. Leitlinien zur Therapie der benignen Struma – G80. Mitt. Deutsch Ges Chir 1998; 3.

[231] Dralle, H, Scheumann, GEW, Hundeshagen, H. et al. Die transsternale zervikomediastinale Primärtumorresektion und Lymphadenektomie beim Schilddrüsenkarzinom. Langenbecks Arch Chir 377:34–44.

[232] Oussoultzoglu, E, Panaro, F, Rosso, E. et al. Use of BiClamp decreased the severity of hypocalcemia after total thyroidectomy compared with ligasure: a prospective study. World J Surg 2008; 32:1968–1973.

[233] Dralle, H, Sekulla, C, Lorenz, K. et al. Intraoperative monitoring of the recurrent larnygeal nerve in thyroid surgery. World J Surg 2008; 32:1358–1366.

[234] Hartel, W, Dralle, H. Leitlinien zur Therapie der benignen Struma. Grundlagen der Chirurgie – G80. Mitt. Deutsch Ges Chir. 1998; Issue 3.

[235] Bauch, J, Bruch, HP, Jähne, J (ed). Behandlungsfehler und Haftpflicht in der Viszeralchirurgie. Springer 2011.

[236] Gagner, M., Inabnet, B. W. III, Biertho, L. Endoscopic thyroidectomy for solitary nodules. Ann Chir 2003; 128:696–701.

[237] Cougard, P, Osmak, L, Esquis, P. et al. Endoscopic thyroidectomy. A preliminary report including 40 patients. Ann Chir 2005; 130:81–85.

[238] Henry, JF, Sebag, F. Lateral endoscopic approach for thyroid and parathyroid surgery. Ann Chir 2006; 131:51–56.

[239] Palazzo, FF, Sebag, F, Henry, JF. Endocrine surgical technique, endoscopic thyroidectomy via the lateral approach. Surg Endosc 2006; 20:339–342.

[240] Sebag, F, Palazzo, FF, Harding, J. et al. Endoscopic lateral approach thyroid obectomy safe evolution from endoscopic parathyroidectomy. World Surg 2006; 30:802–805.

[241] Slotema, ETh, Sebag, F, Henry, JF. What is the Evidence for Endoscopic Thyroidectomy in the Management of Benign Thyroid Disease? Word J Surg 2008; 32(7):1325–1332.

[242] Kitano, H, Fujimura, M, Kinoshita, T. et al. Endoscopic thyroid resection using cutaneous elevation in lieu of insufflation. Surg Endosc 2002; 16:88–91.

[243] Takami, HE, Ikeda, Y. Minimally invasive thyroidectomy. Curr Opin Oncol 2006; 18: 43–47.

[244] Takami, HE, Ikeda, Y. Total endoscopic thyroidectomy. Asian J Surg 2003; 26:82–85.

[245] Ikeda, Y, Takami, H, Sasaki, Y, Takayama, J, Kurihara, H. Are there significant benefits of minimally invasive endoscopic thyroidectomy? World J Surg 2004; 28:1075–1978.

[246] Park, YL, Han, WK, Bae, WG. 100 cases of endoscopic thyroidectomy: breast approach. Surg Laparosc Endosc Percutan Tech 2003; 13:20–25.

[247] Fitz, RH. Perforation inflammation of the vermiform appendix with special reference to its early diagnosis and treatment. Am J Med Sci 1886; 92:321–346.

[248] Addiss, DG, Shaffer, N, Fowler, BS. et al. The epidemiology of appendicitis and appendectomy in the United States. Am J Epidemiol 1990; 132:910–925.

[249] Mc Burney, C. The incision made in the abdominal wall in cases of appendicitis, with a description of a new method of operating. Ann Surg 1894; 20:38–43.

[250] Semm, K. Endoscopic appendectomy. Endoscopy 1983; 15:59–64.

[251] Lippert, H, Koch, A, Marrusch, F, Wolff, S, Gastinger, I. Offene versus laparoskopische Appendektomie. Chirurg 2002; 73:791–798.

[252] Xiaohang, L, Jialin, Z, Lixuan, S. et al. Laparoscopic versus conventionell appendectomy – a meta-analysis of randomized controlled trials. BMC Gastroenterol 2010; 10:129.

[253] Memon, MA. Laparoscopic appendectomy current status. Ann R Coll Surg Eng 1997; 79: 393–402.

[254] Brümmer, S, Sohr, D, Gastmeier, P. Intraabdominal abscesses and laparoscopic versus open appendectomies. Infect Control Hosp Epidemiol 2009; 30:713–715.

[255] Guller, U, Hervey, S, Purves, H. et al. Laparoscopic versus open appendectomy. Ann Surg 2004; 239:43–51.

[256] Spom, E, Petroski, GF, Mancini, GJ. et al. Laparoscopic appendectomy – Is it worth the cost? Trend analysis in the US from 2000 to 2005. J Am Coll Surg 2009; 208:179–185.

[257] Katkhouda, N, Friedländer, MH, Grant, SW, Achanta, KK, Essani, R, Paik, P, Velmahos, G, Campos, G, Mason, R, Mavor, E. Intraabdominal abscess rate after laparoscopic appendectomy. Am J Surg 2000; 180:456–461.

[258] Berry, J, Malt, RA. Appendicitis near its centenary. Ann Surg 1984; 200:567–575.

[259] Schick, KS, Hüttl, TP, Fertmann, JM. et al. A critical analysis of laparoscopic appendectomy: how experience with 1,400 appendectomies allowed innovative treatment to become standard in a university hospital. World J Surg 2008; 32:1406–1413.

[260] Gill, BD, Jenkins, JR. Cost-effective evaluation and treatment of the acute abdomen. Surg Clin North Am 1996; 76:71–82.

[261] Babcock, JR, McKinley, WM. Acute appendicitis: an analysis of 1,662 consecutive cases. Ann Surg 1959; 150:131–141.

[262] Mittelpunkt, A, Nora, PF. Current features in the treatment of acute appendicitis: an analysis of 1,000 cases. Arch Surg 1966; 60:971–975.

[263] Lewis, FR, Holcroft, JW, Boey, J. et al. Appendicitis: a critical review of diagnosis and treatment in 1,000 cases. Arch Surg 1975; 110:677–684.

[264] Silberman, VA. Appendectomy in a large metropolitan hospital. Retrospective analysis of 1,013 cases. Am J Surg 1981; 142:616–618.

[265] Pieper, R, Kager, L, Nasman, P. Acute appendicitis: a clinical study of 1,018 cases of emergency appendectomy. Acta Chir Scand 1982; 148:51–62.

[266] Maxwell, JM, Ragland, JJ. Appendicitis. Improvements in diagnosis and treatment. Am Surg 1991; 57:282–285.

[267] Andersson, RE, Hugander, A, Thulin, AJG. Diagnostic accuracy and perforation rate in appendicitis: association with age and sex of the patient and with appendectomy rate. Eur J Surg 1992; 158:37–41.

[268] Pittman-Waller, VA, Myers, JG, Stewart, RM. et al. Appendicitis why so complicated? Analysis of 5,755 consecutive appendectomies. Am Surg 2000; 66:548–443.

[269] Margenthaler, JA, Walter, E, Katherines, L. et al. Risk factors for adverse outcomes after the surgical treatment of appendicitis in adults. Ann Surg 2003 July; 238(1):59–66.

[270] Putzki, H, Reichert, B. Does measuring of axillorectal temperature difference help in the diagnosis of acute appendicitis? Langenbecks Arch Chir 1988; 373:310–312.

[271] Dixon, JM, Elton, RA, Reiney, JB. et al. DAD: Rectal examination in patients with pain in the right lower quadrant of the abdomen. BMJ 1990; 302:386–388.

[272] Bauch, J, Bruch, HP, Jähne, J (ed). Behandlungsfehler und Haftpflicht in der Viszeralchirurgie. Springer 2011.

[273] Rioux, M. Sonographic detection of the normal and abnormal appendix. Am J Roentgenol 1992; 158:773.

[274] Zielke, A. Appendizitis. Chirurg 2002; 73:782–790.

[275] Dolgin, SE, Beck, AR, Tartter, PI. The risk of perforation when children with possible appendicitis are observed in the hospital. Surg Gynecol Obstet 1992; 175:320.

[276] Graff, L, Radford, MJ, Werne, C. Probability of appendicitis before and after observation. Ann Emerg Med 1991; 20:503.

[277] Thompson, HJ, Jones, PF. Active observation in adults with abdominal pain. Am J Surg 1986; 152:522.

[278] Fink, S, Chadhuri, TK. Risk management in suspective acute appendicitis. Perspectives in health – care risk management 1991; 11:11–4.

[279] Rusnak, RA, Borer, JM. et al. Misdiagnosis of acute appendicitis: common features discovered in cases after litigation. Am J Emergency Med 1994; 12:397–403.

[280] Fingerhut, A, Millar, B, Borrie, F. Laparoscopic versus open appendectomy: time to decide: World J Surg 1999; 23:835–845.

[281] Frizelle, FA, Hanna, GB. Pelvic abscess following laparoscopic appendectomy [letter]. Surg Endosc 1996; 10:947–948.

[282] Golub, R, Siddiqui, F, Pohl, D. Laparoscopic versus open appendectomy: a metaanalysis. J Am Coll Surg 1998; 186:545–553.

[283] Horwitz, JR, Custer, MD, May, BH, Mehall, JR, Lally, KP. Should laparoscopic appendectomy be avoided for complicated appendicitis in children? J Pediatr Surg 1997; 32:1601–1603.

[284] Klingler, A, Henle, KP, Beller, S, Rechner, J, Zerz, A, Wetscher, GJ, Szinicz, G. Laparoscopic appendectomy does not change the incidence of postoperative infectious complications. Am J Surg 1998; 175:232–235.

[285] Koch, A, Marusch, F, Gastinger, I. Appendizitis: Wann laparoskopisch und wann konventionell operieren? Chir Gastroenterol 2000; 16:126–130.

[286] Nguyen, DB, Silen, W, Hodin, RA. Appendectomy in the pre- and post-laparoscopic eras. J Gastrointest Surg 1999; 3:67–73.

[287] Ortega, AE, Hunter, JG, Peters, JH, Swanstrom, LL, Schirmer, BA. Prospective, randomised comparison of laparaoscopic appendectomy with open appendectomy. Am J Surg 1995; 169:208–212.

[288] Paik, PS, Towson, JA, Anthone, GJ, Ortega, AE, Simons, AJ, Beart, RW. Intraabdominal abscesses following laparoscopic and open appendectomies. J Gastrointest Surg 1997; 1: 188–192.

[289] Reid, RI, Dobbs, BR, Frizelle, FA. Risk factors for post-appendectomy intraabdominal abscess. Aust NZ J Surg 1999; 69; 373–374.

[290] Reiertsen, O, Trondsen, E, Bakka, A, Andersen, OK, Larsen, S, Rosseland, AR. Prospective nonrandomized study of conventional versus laparoscopic appendectomy. World J Surg 1994; 18:411–416.

[291] Tang, E, Ortega, AE, Anthone, GJ, Beart, RWJ. Intraabdominal abscesses following laparoscopic and open appendectomies. Surg Endosc 1996; 10:327–328.

[292] Tate, JJT, Chung, SCS, Dawson, J, Leong, HT, Chan, A, Lau, WY, Li, AKC. Conventional versus laparoscopic surgery for acute appendicitis. Br. J Surg 1993; 80:761–764.

[293] Sauerland, S, Lefering, R, Neugebauer, EA. Laparoscopic versus open surgery for suspected appendicitis (Cochrane Review) [In Process Citation]. Cochrane Database Syst Rev 2002; CD001546.

[294] Kazemier, G, Hof in't, KH, Saad, S. et al. Securing the appendiceal stump in laparoscopic appendectomy: evidence for routine stapling? Surg Endosc 2006; 20:1473–1476.

[295] Meyer-Marcotty, W, Plarre, I. Die chronische Appendizitis. Langenbecks Archives of Surgery 1986; 369:187.

[296] Becker, K, Hofler, H. Pathophysiologie der Appendizitis. Chirurg 2002; 73:777–781.

[297] Liang, M, Lo, K, Marks, JL. Stump appendicitis: a comprehensive review of literature. Am Surg 2006; 72:162–166.

[298] Walsh, DC, Roediger, WE. Stump appendicitis – a potential problem after laparoscopic appendectomy. Surg Laparoscop Endosc 1997; 7:357–358.

[299] Bruce, J, Krukowski, ZH, Al-Khairy, G. et al. Systematic review of the definition and measurement of anastomotic leak after gastrointestinal surgery. Br J Surg 2001; 88:1157–1168.

[300] Welsch, T, von Frankenberg, M, Büchler, MW. et al. Diagnostik und Definition der Nahtin-suffizienz aus chirurgischer Sicht. Chirurg 2001; 82:48–55.

[301] Heald, RJ, Leicester, R. The low stapled anastomoses. Br J Surg 1981; 68:333.

[302] Karanjia, N, Corder, A, Bearn, P. et al. Leakage from stapled low anastomoses after total mesorectal excision for carcinoma of the rectum. Br J Surg 1994; 81:1224.

[303] Pakkastie, T, Luukkonen, P, Järvinen, HJ. Anastomotic leakage after anterior resection of the rectum. Eur J Surg 1994; 160:293.

[304] Farke, S, Gögler, H. Anastomoseninsuffizienz nach kontinenzerhaltenden Rektumresektionen. Coloproctology 2006; 22: no 5.

[305] Järvinen, HJ, Luukkonen, P. Sphincter saving surgery for rectal carcinoma. Ann Chir Gyne-col 1991; 80:14–8.

[306] Kessler, H, Hermanek, Jr. P, Wiebelt, H. Operative mortality in carcinoma of the rectum. Results of the German Multicentre Study. Int J Colorect Dis 1993; 8:158–66.

[307] Martens, MF, Hendriks, T. Postoperative changes in collagen synthesis in intestinal anas-tomoses of the rat: differences between small and large bowel. Gut 1991; 32(12):1482–1487.

[308] Golub, R, Golub, RW, Cantu, R, Stein, HD. A multivariate analysis of factors contributing to leakage of intestinal anastomoses. Am Coll Surg 1997; 184:361.

[309] Mäkelä, JT, Kiviniemi, H, Laitinen, S. Risk factors for anastomotic leakage after left-sided colorectal resection with rectal anastomoses. Dis Colon Rectum 2003; 46:653.

[310] Kingham, TP, Pachter, HL. Colonic anastomotic risk factors, diagnosis and treatment. J Am Coll Surg 2009; 208(2):269–278.

[311] Konishi, I, Watanabe, T, Kishimoto, J, Nagawa, H. Risk factors for anastomotic leakage after surgery for colorectal cancer: results of prospective Surveillance. J Am Coll Surg 2006; 203(3):439–44.

[312] Biondo, S, Parés, D, Kreisler, E. et al. Anastomotic dehiscence after resection and primary anastomoses in left-sided colonic emergencies. Dis Colon Rectum 2005; 48(12):2272–2280.

[313] Vignali, A, Fazio, VW, Lavery, IC. et al. Factors associated with the occurrence of leaks in stapled rectal anastomoses: a review of 1,014 patients. J Am Coll Surg 1997; 185(2):105–113.

[314] Clinical Outcomes of Surgical Therapy Study Group. A comparison of laparoscopically assisted and open colectomy for colon cancer. N Engl J Med 2004; 350(20):2050–2059.

[315] Docherty, JG, Mc Gregor, JR, Akyol, AM, Murray, GD, Galloway, DJ. West of Scotland and Highland Anastomoses Study Group. Comparison of manually constructed and stapled anastomoses in colorectal surgery. Ann Surg 1995; 221(2):176–184.

[316] Lustosa, SA, Matos, D, Atallah, AN, Casto, AA. Stapled versus handsewn methods for col-orectal anastomoses surgery. Cochrane Database Syst Rev. 2001; (3):DC003144.

[317] Patankar, SK, Larach, SW, Ferrara, A. et al. Prospective comparison of laparoscopic vs. open resections for colorectal adenocarcinoma over a ten-year period. Dis Colon Rectum 2003; 46(5):601–611.

[318] Beard, JD, Nicholson, ML, Sayers, RD, Lloyd, D, Everson, NW. Intraoperative air testing of colorectal anastomoses: a prospective randomized trial. Br J Surg 1990; 77(10):1095–1097.

[319] Telem, DA, Chin, EH, Nguyen, SQ. Risk factors for anastomotic leak following colorectal surgery. Arch Surg 2010; 145(4):371–376.

[320] Clark, MA, Plamk, LD, Hill, GL. Wound healing associated with severe surgical illness. World J Surg 2000; 24:648.

[321] Jensen, JA, Goodson, W. Hopf, HW, Hunt, TK. Cigarette smoking decreases tissue oxygen. Arch Surg 1991; 126:1131.

[322] Jorgensen, LN, Kallehave, F, Christensen, E, Siana, JE, Gottrup, F. Less collagen production in smokers. Surgery 1998; 123:450.

[323] Lahmann, C, Bergemann, J, Harrison, G, Young, AR. Matrix metalloproteinase-1 and skin ageing in smokers. Lancet 2001; 357:935.

[324] Sorensen, LT, Jorgensen, T, Kirkeby, LT, Skovdal, J, Vennits, B, Wille-Jorgensen, P. Smoking and alcohol abuse are major risk factors for anastomotic leakage in colorectal surgery. Br J Surg 1999; 86:927.

[325] Polat, A, Nayci, A, Polat, G, Aksoyek, S. Dexamethasone down-regulated endothelial expression of intercellular adhesion molecule and impairs healing of bowel anastomoses. Eur J Surg 2002; 168:500.

[326] Valente, JF, Hricik, D, Weigel, K. et al. Comparison of sirolimus vs. mycophenolate mofetil on surgical complications and wound healing in adult kidney transplantation. Am J Transplant 2003; 3:1128.

[327] Alves, A, Panis, Y, Trancart, D, Regimbeau, JM, Pocard, M, Valleur, P. Factors associated with clinically significant anastomotic leakage after large bowel resection: multivariate analysis of 707 patients. World J Surg 2002; 26:499.

[328] Ahrendt, GM, Gardner, K, Barbul, A. Loss of colonic structural collagen impairs healing during intra-abdominal sepsis. Arch Surg 1994; 129:1179.

[329] Wolf, AM, Henne-Bruns, D. Anastomoseninsuffizienz im Gastrointestinaltrakt. Chirurg 2002; 73:394–407.

[330] Jonsson, K, Jensen, A, Goodson, WH, Scheuenstuhl, H, West, J, Hopf, HW. Hunt, TK. Tissue oxygenation, anaemia and perfusion in relation to wound healing in surgical patients. Ann Surg 1991; 214:605.

[331] Senagore, A, Milsom, JW, Walshaw, RK, Dunstan, R, Mazier, WP, Chaudry, IC. Intramural pH: a quantitative measurement for predicting colorectal anastomotic healing. Dis Colon Rectum 1990; 33:175.

[332] Stumpf, M, Klinge, U, Mertens, PR. Prognostische Faktoren. Chirurg 2004; 75:1056–1062.

[333] Carty, NJ, Keating, J, Campbell, J, Karanjia, N, Heald, RJ. Prospective audit of an extramucosal technique for intestinal anastomoses. Br J Surg 1991; 78:1439.

[334] Leslie, A, Steele, RJ. The interrupted seromucosal anastomoses – still the gold standard. Colorectal Dis 2003; 5:362.

[335] Ferri, EL, Law, S, Wong, KH. et al. The influence of technical complications on postoperative outcome and survival after esophagectomy. Annals of Surgical Oncology 2006; 13/4: 557–564.

[336] Millikan, KW, Silverstein, J, Hart, V. et al. A 15-year review of esophagectomy for carcinoma of the esophagus and cardia. Arch Surg 1995; 130:617–24.

[337] Ellis, Jr. FH, Heatly, GJ, Krasna, MJ, Williamson, WA, Balogh, K. Esophagogastrectomy for carcinoma of the esophagus and cardia: a comparison of findings and results after standard resection in three consecutive eight-year intervals with improved staging criterias. J Thorac Cardiovasc Surg 1997; 113:836–846.

[338] Thomas, P, Doddoli, C, Lienne, P. et al. Changing patterns and surgical results in adenocarcinoma of the oesophagus. Br J Surg 1997; 84:119–25.

[339] Hagen, JA, De Meester, SR, Peters, JH, Chandrasoma, P, De Meester, TR. Curative resection for esophageal adenocarcinoma: analysis of 100 en bloc esophagectomies. Ann Surg 2001; 234:520–30.

[340] Law, S, Kwong, DI, Kwok, KF. et al. Improvement in treatment results and long-term survival of patients with esophageal cancer: impact of chemoradiation and change in treatment strategy. Ann Surg 2003; 238:339–47.

[341] Ando, N, Ozawa, S, Kitagawa, Y, Shinozawa, Y, Kitajima, M. Improvement in the results of surgical treatment of advanced squamous esophageal carcinoma during 15 consecutive years. Ann Surg 2000; 232:225–32.

[342] Jamieson, GG, Mathew, G, Lüdemann, R. et al. Postoperative mortality following esophagectomy and problems in reporting its rate. Br Surg 2004; 91:943–947.

[343] Orringer, MB, Marshall, B, Iannettoni, MD. Transhiatal esophagectomy: clinical experience and refinements. Ann Surg 1999; 230:392–400.

[344] van Sandick, JW, van Lanschot, JJ, ten Kate, FJ, Tijssen, JG, Obertop, H. Indicators of prognosis after transhiatal esophageal resection without thoracotomy for cancer. J Am Coll Surg 2002; 194(1):28–36.

[345] Hofstetter, W, Swisher, SG, Correa, AM. et al. Treatment outcomes of resected esophageal cancer. Ann Surg 2002; 236:376–84.

[346] Karl, RC, Schreiber, R, Boulware, D, Baker, S, Coppola, D. Factors affecting morbidity, mortality, and survival in patients undergoing Ivor Lewis esophagogastrectomy. Ann Surg 2000; 231:635–43.

[347] Siewert, JR. Oesophaguskarzinom. Onkologe 2007; 13:949–960.

[348] Giuli, R, Gignoux, M. Treatment of carcinoma of the esophagus. Retrospective study of 2,400 patients. Ann Surg 1980; 192:44–52.

[349] Chasseray, VM, Kiroff, GK, Buard, JL, Launois, BL. Cervical on thoracic anastomoses for esophagectomy for carcinoma. Surg Gynec Obstetrics 1989; 169:55–62.

[350] Clark, GWB, Peter, JH, Ireland, AP. et al. Nodal metastasis and sites of recurrence after en-bloc esophagectomy for adenocarcinoma. Ann Thorac Surg 1994; 58:646–654.

[351] Hulscher, JBF, van Sandick, JW, Offerhaus, GJA. et al. Prospective analysis of the diagnostic yield of extended en bloc resection for adenocarcinoma of the esophagus or gastric cardia. Br J Surg 2001; 88:715–719.

[352] Luketich, JD, Alvelo-Rivera, M, Buenaventura, PO, Christie, NA, Mc Caughan, JS, Little, VR. et al. Minimally-invasive esophagectomy. Outcomes in 222 patients. Ann Surg 2003; 238: 486–494.

[353] Palanivelu, C, Prakash, A, Senthilkumar, R, Senthilnathan, P, Parthasarathi, R, Rajan, S. et al. Minimally invasive esophagectomy: thorascopc mobilization of the esophagus and mediastinal lymphadenectomy in prone position – experience of 130 patients. J Am Coll Surg 2006; 203:7–16.

[354] Ben-David, K, Rossidis, G, Zlotecki, RA. et al. Minimally invasive esophagectomy is safe and effective following neoadjuvant chemoradiation therapy. Ann Surg Oncol 2011; 18: 3324–3329.

[355] Murthy, SC, Law, S, Whooley, BP. et al. A trial fibrillation after esophagectomy is a marker for postoperative morbidity and mortality. J Thorac Cardiovasc Surg 2003; 126(4): 1162–1167.

[356] von Rahden, BHA, Stein, HJ, Siewert, JR. Barrett's Esophagus and Barrett's Cancer. Curr Oncol Rep 2003; 5:203–209.

[357] Siewert, JR, Hölscher, AH, Becker, K. et al. Cardia Cancer: Attempt at a therapeutically relevant classification. Chirurg 1987; 58:25–32.

[358] Sasako, M, Sano, T, Yamamoto, S. et al. Left thoracoabdominal approach versus abdominal-transhiatal approach for gastric. Cancer of the cardia or subcardia: A randomized controlled trial. Lancet Oncol 2006; 7:644–651.

[359] Schneider, PM, Müller, MK, Schiesser, M. Chirurgische Therapiestrategien beim Oesophagus-Magenkarzinom. Gastroenterologe 2009; 4:209–223.

[360] Bozzetti, F, Marubini, E, Bonfanti, G. et al. Total versus subtotal gastrectomy: Surgical morbidity and mortality rates in a multicenter Italian randomized trail. The Italian Gastrointestinal Tumor Study Group. Ann Surg 1997; 226:613–620.

[361] Gouzi, JL, Huguier, M, Fagniez, PL. et al. Total versus subtotal gastrectomy for adenocarcinoma of the gastric antrum. A French prospective controlled study. Ann Surg 1989; 209: 162–166.

[362] Kitano, S, Iso, Y, Moriyama, M, Sugimachi, K. Laparoscopy-assisted Billroth I gastrectomy. Surg Laparosc Endosc Percutan Tech 1994; 4:146–148.

[363] Kitano, S, Shiraishi, N, Fuji, K. et al. A randomized controlled trial comparing open vs laparoscopy-assisted distal gastrectomy for the treatment of early gastric cancer. An interim report. Surgery 2002; 131 (1 Suppl): 5306.

[364] Kitawaga, Y, Kitano, S, Kubota, T. et al. Minimally invasive surgery for gastric cancer - toward a confluence of two major streams: A review. Gastric Cancer 2005; 8:103–110.

[365] Ohgami, M, Otani, Y, Kumai, K. et al. Curative laparoscopic surgery for early gastric cancer. Five years experience. World J Surg 1999; 23:187–192.

[366] Jähne, J. Chirurgische Komplikationen. In: Meyer, HJ, Buhr, HJ, Wilke, H (ed). Management des distalen Oesophagus- und Magenkarzinoms. Springer Berlin 2004; p. 325–332.

[367] Hyodo, M, Hosaya, Y, Hirashima, Y. et al. Minimum leakage rate (0,5%) of stapled esophago-jejunostomy with sacrifice of a small part of the jejunum after total gastrectomy in 390 consecutive patients. Dig Surg 2007; 24:269–272.

[368] Siewert, JR, Stein, HJ, Bartels, H. Insuffizienzen nach Anastomosen im Bereich des oberen Gastrointestinaltraktes. Chirurg 2004; 75:1063–1070.

[369] Tonouchi, H, Mohri, Y, Tanaka, K. et al. Diagnostic sensitivity of contrast swallow for leakage after gastric resection. World J Surg 2006; 31:128–131.

[370] Meyer, HJ, Sauer, P. Postoperative Probleme nach Magenresektion oder Gastrektomie und Pankreasresektion. Gastroenterologe 2009; 4:437.445.

[371] Hohenberger, W. Offene Rektumchirurgie. Chirurg 2007; 78:739–747.

[372] Matthiesen, P, Hallböök, O, Rutegard, J. et al. Defunctioning stoma reduces symptomatic anastomotic leakage after low anterior resection of the rectum for cancer: a randomized multicenter trial. Ann Surg 2007; 246(2):207–14.

[373] Hida, J, Yasutomi, M, Maruyama, T. et al. Lymph node metastases detected in the mesorectum distal to carcinoma of the rectum by the clearing method: justification of total mesorectal excision. J Am Coll Surg 1997; 184:584–8.

[374] Heald, RJ, Husband, EM, Ryall, RD. The mesorectum in the rectal cancer surgery – the clue to pelvic recurrence? Br J Surg 1982; 69:613–6.

[375] Enker, WE, Merchant, N, Cohen, AM. et al. Safety and efficacy of low anterior resection for rectal cancer: 681 consecutive cases from a specialty service. Ann Surg 1999; 230:544–54.

[376] Schiedeck, THK. et al. Laparoscopic surgery for the cure of colorectal cancer. Dis Colon Rectum 2000; 431–438.

[377] Fowler, DL, White, SA. Laparoscopic-assisted sigmoid resection. Surg Laparosc Endosc 1991; 1:183–8.

[378] Breukink, S, Pierie, J, Wiggers, T. Laparoscopic versus open total mesorectal excision for rectal cancer. Cochrane Database Syst Rev 2006; CD005200.

[379] Lamme, B, Boermaster, MA, Reitsma, JB. et al. Metaanalysis of relaparotomy for secondary peritonitis. Br J Surg 2002; 89:1516–1524.

[380] Bartels, H. Spezielle Gesichtspunkte postoperativer Komplikationen in der Viszeralchirurgie. Chirurg 2009; 80:780–789.

[381] Willis, S, Stumpf, M. Insuffizienzen nach Eingriffen am unteren Gastrointestinaltrakt. Chirurg 2000; 75:1071–1078.

[382] Goligher, JC, Graham, NG, Drukal, FT. Anastomotic dehiscence after anterior resection of rectum and sigmoid. Br J Surg 1970; 57109–19.

[383] Rexer, M, Ditterich, D. Rupprecht, H. Vakuumtherapie bei kolorektaler Anastomoseninsuffizienz. Coloproctology 2004; 26:285–290.

[384] Barth, U. Vorkommnismeldungen bei Klammernahtinstrumenten. Chirurg 2009; 80:735–740.

[385] Ockert, D, Bergert, H, Knopke, R, Saeger, HD. Das akute Abdomen. Gynäkologe 2003; 35:336–339.

[386] De Dombal, FT. The OMGE acute abdominal pain survey. Progress report, 1986. Scand J Gastroenterol 1988; 23 (144):36–42.

[387] Miettinen, P, Pasanen, P, Lahtinen, J, Alhava, E. Acute abdominal pain in adults. Ann Chir Gynaecol 1996; 85:5–9.

[388] Lankisch, PG, Mahlke, R, Lübbers, H. Zertifizierte medizinische Fortbildung: Das akute Abdomen aus internistischer Sicht. Dtsch Ärztebl 2006; 103: A-2179/B-1884/C-1821.

[389] De Dombal, FT. Diagnosis of acute abdominal pain. Edinburgh, London, Melbourne, New York: Churchill Livingstone 1991.

[390] Kersting, S, Saeger, HD. Akutes Abdomen. In: Bauch, J, Bruch, HP, Heberer, J, Jähne, J. Behandlungsfehler und Haftpflicht in der Viszeralchirurgie. 2011; 323–334.

[391] Schwerk, WB. Ultrasound first in acute appendix? Unnecessary laparotomies can often be avoided. Muench Med Wschr 2000; 142:29–32.

[392] Manner, M, Stickel, W. Diagnostik bei Verdacht auf Appendicitis – Lässt sich eine Appendicitis sonographisch ausschließen? Chirurg 2001; 72:1036–1042.

[393] Gwynn, LK. The Diagnosis of acute appendicitis: clinical assessment versus computed tomography evaluation. J Emerg Med 21:119–123.

[394] Klempa, I. Zeitgemäße Therapie der komplizierten Appendizitis. Chirurg 2002; 73:799–804.

[395] Cope, VZ. The diagnosis of the acute abdomen in rhyme. Lewis, HK. London 1947.

[396] Schein, M. Schein's Common sense emergency abdominal surgery. Springer, Berlin, Heidelberg, New York, 2000.

[397] Mulier, S, Penninckx, F, Verwaest, C, Filez, L, Aerts, R, Fieuws, S. et al. Factors affecting mortality in generalized postoperative peritonitis: multivariate analysis in 96 patients. World J Surg. 2003; 27:379–84.

[398] Ivatury, RR, Nallathambi, M, Rao, PM, Rohman, M, Stahl, WM. Open management of the septic abdomen: therapeutic and prognostic considerations based on APACHE II. Crit Care Med. 1989; 17:511–7.

[399] Holzheimer, RG, Gathof, B. Re-operation for complicated secondary peritonitis – how to identify patients at risk for persistent sepsis. Eur J Med Res 2003; 8:125–34.

[400] Tsiotos, GG, Luque-de Leon, E, Soreide, JA, Bannon, MP, Zietlow, SP, Baerga-Varela, Y. et al. Management of necrotizing pancreatitis by repeated operative necrosectomy using a zipper technique. Am J Surg 1998; 175:91–8.

[401] Pacelli, F, Doglietto, GB, Alfieri, S, Piccioni, E, Sgadari, A, Gui, D. et al. Prognosis in intraabdominal infections. Multivariate analysis on 604 patients. Arch Surg 1996; 131:641–5.

[402] Dellinger, RP. Cardiovascular management of septic shock. Crit Care Med. 2003; 31:946–55.

[403] Strobel, C, Büchler, MW. Chirurgische Therapie der Peritonitis. Chirurg 2011; 82:242–248.

[404] Fahrtmann, EH, Schoffel, U. Principles and limitations of operative management of intraabdominal infections. World J Surg 1990; 14:210–217.

[405] Wacha, H, Hau, T, Dittmer, R, Ohmann, C. Risk factors associated with intraabdominal infections: a prospective multicenter study. Peritonitis Study Group. Langenbecks Arch Surg 1999; 384:24–32.

[406] Levy, MM. et al. 2001 SCCM/ESICM/ACCP/ATS/SIS International Sepsis Definitions Conference. Crit Care Med 2003; 31:1250–1256.

[407] Knaus, WA, Draper, EA, Wagner, DP, Zimmermann, JE. APACHE II: a severity of disease classification system. Crit Care Med. 1985; 13:818–829.

[408] Marshall, JC. et al. Multiple organ dysfunction score: a reliable descriptor of a complex clinical outcome. Crit Care Med 1995; 23:1638–1652.

[409] Vincent, JL. et al. The SOFA (Sepsis-related Organ Failure Assessment) score to describe organ dysfunction/failure. On behalf of the Working Group of Sepsis-Related Problems of the European Society of Intensive Care Medicine. Intensive Care Med. 1996; 22:707–710.

[410] Christou, NV, Barie, PS, Dellinger, EP, Waymack, JP, Stone, HH. Surgical Infection Society intra-abdominal infection study. Prospective evaluation of management techniques and outcome. Arch Surg 1993; 128:193–198.

[411] Koperna, T, Schulz, F. Prognosis and treatment of peritonitis. Do we need new scoring systems? Arch Surg 1996; 131:180–186.

[412] Gooszen, AW. et al. Operative treatment of acute complications of diverticular disease: primary or secondary anastomosis after sigmoid resection. Eur J Surg 2001; 167:35–39.

[413] van Westreenen, M. et al. Influence of peroperative lavage solutions on peritoneal defence mechanisms in vitro. Eur J Surg 1999; 165:1066–1071.

[414] Hallerback, B, Andersson, C, Englund, N. et al. A prospective randomized study of continuous peritoneal lavage postoperatively in the treatment of purulent peritonitis. Surg Gynecol Obstet 1986; 163:433–436.

[415] Pichlmayr, R, Lehr, I, Pahlow, J, Guthy, E. Postoperative continuous open dorsoventral abdominal lavage in severe forms of peritonitis. Chirurg 1983; 54:299–305.

[416] Bartels, H, Barthlen, W, Siewert, JR. The therapeutic results of programmed relaparotomy in diffuse peritonitis. Chirurg 1992; 63:174–180.

[417] Schein, M. Planned reoperations and open management in critical intra-abdominal infections: prospective experience in 52 cases. World J Surg 1991; 15:537–545.

[418] Hau, T, Ohmann, C, Wolmershausen, A. et al. Planned relaparotomy vs relaparotomy on demand in the treatment of intra-abdominal infections. The Peritonitis Study Group of the Surgical Infection Society-Europe. Arch Surg 1995; 130:1193–1196.

[419] Teichmann, W, Wittmann, DH, Andreone, PA. Scheduled reoperations (Etappenlavage) for diffuse peritonitis. Arch Surg 1986; 121:147–152.

[420] Mughal, MM, Bancewicz, J, Irving, MH. Laparostomy: a technique for the management of intractable intra-abdominal sepsis. Br J Surg 1986; 73:253–259.

[421] Bosscha, K, Hulstaert, PF, Visser, MR., van Vroonhoven, ThJMV, van der Werken, Chr. Open management of the abdomen and planned reoperations, in severe bacterial peritonitis. Eur J Surg 2000; 166:44–49.

[422] Schein, M. Management of severe intra-abdominal infection. Surg Annu 1992; 24 Pt 1: 47–68.

[423] Büchler, MW, Baer, HU, Brugger, LE. et al. Surgical therapy of diffuse peritonitis: debridement and intraoperative extensive lavage. Chirurg 1997; 68:811–815.

[424] Lamme, B. et al. Meta-analysis of relaparotomy for secondary peritonitis. Br J Surg 2002; 89:1516–1524.

[425] Lamme, B, Mahler, CW, van Till, JWC. et al. Relaparotomie bei sekundärer Peritonitis. Chirurg 2005; 76:856–867.

[426] Hong, JJ. et al. Prospective study of the incidence and outcome of intra-abdominal hypertension and the abdominal compartment syndrome. Br J Surg 2002; 89:591–596.

[427] Henne-Bruns, D, Löhnert, M. Aktueller Stand zu Diagnostik und nicht operativen Therapie des Dünndarmileus. Chirurg 2000; 71:503–509.

[428] Bruch, HP. Ileus-Krankheit. Chirurg 1989; 60:198–202.

[429] Mirkovitch, V, Cobo, F, Robinson, JWL, Menge, H, Combo, SZ. Morphology and function of the dog ileum after mechanical occlusion. Clin Sci Med 1976; 50:123.

[430] Shields, R. The absorption and secretion of fluid and electrolytes in the obstructed bowel. Br J Surg 1965; 52:774.

[431] Sykes, PA, Boulter, KH, Schofield, PF. Small bowel microflora in acute intestinal obstruction and Crohn's disease. Br J Surg 1974; 52:774.

[432] Roscher, R, Frank, R, Baumann, A, Beger, HG. Chirurgische Behandlungsergebnisse beim mechanischen Dünndarmileus. Chirurg 1991; 62:614.

[433] Renzulli, P, Krähenbühl, L, Sadowski, C, Al-Adili, F. et al. Moderne diagnostische Strategie beim Ileus. Zentralbl Chir 1998; 123:1334.

[434] Kukor, JS, Dent, TL. Small intestinal obstruction. In: Nelson, RL, Nyhus, LM. (eds). Surgery of the small intestine. Appleton u. Lange 1987; Norwalk, p 267.

[435] Mucha, Jr. P. Small intestinal obstruction. Surg Clin North Am 1987; 67:597–620.

[436] Miller, G, Boman, J, Shrier, I. et al. Etiology of small bowel obstruction. Am J Surg 2000; 180:33–36.

[437] Cox, MR, Gunn, IF, Eastman, M.C. et al. The operative aetiology and types of adhesions causing small bowel obstruction. Aust NZ J Surg 1993; 63:848–852.

[438] Ellis, H, Moran, BJ, Thompson, JN. et al. Adhesion-related hospital readmissions after abdominal and pelvic surgery: a retrospective cohort study. Lancet 1999; 353:1476–1480.

[439] Landercasper, J, Cogbill, TH, Merry, WH. et al. Long-term outcome after hospitalization for small bowel obstruction. Arch Surg. 1993; 128:765–770.

[440] Miller, G, Boman, J, Shrier, I. et al. Natural history of patients with adhesive small bowel obstruction. Br J Surg. 2000; 87:1240–1247.

[441] Fevang, BT, Fevang, J, Lie, SA. et al. Long-term prognosis after operation for adhesive small bowel obstruction. Ann Surg. 2004; 240:193–201.

[442] Barkan, H, Webster, S, Ozeran, S. Factors predicting the recurrence of adhesive small bowel obstruction. Am J Surg. 1995; 170:361–365.

[443] Post, S, Schuster, KL. Verlassenes, Bewährtes und Aktuelles zu operativer Dünndarmileus-Therapie. Chirurg 2000; 71:524–531.

[444] Cox, MR, Gunn, JF, Eastman, MC. et al. The safety and duration of non-operative treatment for adhesive small bowel obstruction. Aust NZ J Surg. 1993; 63:367.

[445] Barnett, WO, Petro, AB, Williamson, JW. A current appraisal of problems with gangrenous bowel. Ann Surg 1976; 183:653.

[446] Becker, WF. Acute adhesive ileus. A study of 412 cases with particular reference to the abuse of tube decompression in treatment. Surg. Gynecol. Obstet 1952; 95:472.

[447] Hofstetter, SR. Acute adhesive obstruction of small intestine. Surg. Gynecol. Obstet. 1981; 152:141.

[448] Silen, W. Strangulation obstruction of the small intestine. Arch. Surg. 1962; 85:137.

[449] Ibrahim, JM, Wolodiger, E, Sussman, B. et al. Laparoscopic management of acute small bowel obstruction. Surg. Endosc. 1996; 10:1014–1015.

[450] Leon, EL, Metzger, A, Tsiotos, G. G. et al. Laparoscopic management of small bowel obstruction. Indications and outcome. J Gastrointest 1998; Surg 2:132–140.

[451] Kreis, ME, Jauch, KW. Ileus aus chirurgischer Sicht. Chirurg 2006; 77:883–888.

[452] Freitag, M, Ludwig, K. et al. Klinische und bildgebende Aspekte des Gallensteinileus. Chirurg 1998; 69: 265–269.

[453] Hildebrandt, J, Herrmann, U, Dietrich, H. Der Gallensteinileus und ein Bericht aus 104 Beobachtungen. Chirurg 1990; 61:392.

[454] Lock, G. Akute mesenteriale Ischämie – häufig übersehen und häufig fatal. In: Medizinische Klinik 2002; 97:402–409.

[455] Eckstein, H. Die akute Mesenterialischämie. Chirurg 2003; 74:419–431.

[456] van Geloven, AW, Biesheuvel, TH, Luitse, JSK, Hoitsma, HFW, Obertop, H. Hospital admissions of patients aged over 80 years with acute abdominal complaints. Eur J Surg 2000; 166:866–871.

[457] Lembcke, B. Pathophysiologie der gastrointestinalen Ischämie und deren klinische Problematik. Chir Gastroenterologie 2002; 6:529–539.

[458] Boley, SJ, Feinstein, FR, Sammartano, R. et al. New concepts in the management of emboli of the superior mesenteric artery. Surg Gynecol Obstet 1981; 153:561–9.

[459] Ritz, JP, Runkel, N, Berger, G. et al. Prognosefaktoren des Mesenterialinfarktes. Zentralbl. Chir. 1997; 122:332–8.

[460] Walter, P, Lindemann, W, Koch, B, Feifel, G. Der akute Mesenterialinfarkt. Klinikarzt 1992; 21:4457–463.

[461] Paes, E, Vollmar, J.F, Hutschenreiter, S, Schoenberg, M.H, Schölzel, E. Diagnostik und Therapie des akuten Mesenterialinfarkts. Chir. Gastroenterologie 1990; 6:473–480.

[462] Inderbitzi, R, Wagner, HE, Seiler, C. et al. Acute mesenteric ischaemia. Eur J. Surg 1992; 158:123–6.

[463] Bjorck, M. et al. Die akute mesenteriale Ischämie. Chirurg 2003; 74:419–431.

[464] Wadman, M, Syk, I, Elmstahl, S. Survival after operations for ischaemic bowel disease. Eur J Surg 2000; 166:872–877.

3 Retained surgical foreign bodies

3.1 Introduction

Not infrequently, foreign bodies are left behind unintentionally after surgery has finished. If this happens, it automatically leads to malpractice claims. This issue most frequently occurs in the field of abdominal or gynecological surgery, but it affects other medical disciplines as well. There are few publications on the topic, not in the least out of fear of liability claims. However, because it encompasses so much, the issue is of exceptional importance.

3.2 The issue of retained surgical foreign bodies

It is a nightmare for both surgeon and patient, if a foreign body is accidentally left behind after surgery has finished. Due to an understandable fear of medical-legal consequences and reputation damage, there is a certain hesitance in publishing on this aspect of patient safety. Rough estimates from insurance companies in the USA assume a rate of one case for every 1,500 operations, which is larger than the number given in the mainstream medical literature [1]. The issues of retained surgical foreign bodies (RSFBs) have existed ever since humans first performed surgery and continues to be a significant problem. Other publications estimate the incidence of RSFBs in the USA at 0.3–1.0 per 1,000 abdominal procedures [2]. When looking at all surgical specialisms together, one RSFB event occurs for every 3,000 operations. For intra-abdominal surgery by itself, the number is one in every 1,000 to 1,500 operations [3, 4].

A study from a medical malpractice insurance company reported 40 cases over a seven-year period, which corresponds to about 1% of all claims [5]. A retrospective review of data from a statewide insurance company in Massachusetts listed 67 cases of malpractice claims resulting from retained sponges or other surgical materials.

The study mentioned above shows that abdominal surgical procedures were responsible for 55% of retained compresses and sponges and 16% was related to vaginal hysterectomy. In 76% of cases, the total number of sponges and compresses was checked and erroneously deemed complete. In 10% of cases, no counting at all was done [6]. Interestingly, in three out of 29 cases, an intraoperative radiological examination to detect X-ray-opaque objects gave a false negative result [5]. Numerous technical terms have been applied to different types of retained surgical objects. For retained sponges and towels, the most frequently used terms include soft tissue textiloma, gossypiboma (from the Latin "gossypium", meaning "cotton" and Swahili "boma" meaning "place of concealment") [7], muslinoma (named after cotton cloth, imported from the city of Mosul in Iraq) [8], and gauzoma [9].

There are no specialized medical terms for retained surgical instruments and needles. Mouhsine et al. proposed a classification of RSFB into exudative (early) and delayed (fibrinous) forms [10, 11]. Retained surgical foreign bodies may harm patients and can result in serious professional and medical-legal consequences [7, 12, 13].

Since it often causes non-specific and highly variable symptoms, recognizing an RSFB presents physicians with a serious diagnostic problem. Frequently, patients only complain about nonspecific abdominal pain. Quite often, an extended period of time elapses between the end of surgery and the onset of clinically recognizable symptoms, especially if retained compresses and sponges were sterile [14, 15]. Most modern surgical textiles are inert and do not take part in biochemical reactions. Usually, they induce intraabdominal adhesions, whereby the foreign body is encapsulated in connective tissue [13, 16]. Acute, early clinical symptoms often develop in cases of exudative reactions or in conjunction with bacterial infections. These symptoms usually are consistent with abdominal or pelvic sepsis, often accompanied by the formation of fistulas, or invasion of intraabdominal hollow viscera. In fact, an RSFB may even be eliminated from the body via natural ways [17–23, 17]. Larger, metallic foreign bodies are often discovered in an earlier stage, since they can be easily identified in medical imaging. Although they may rapidly cause organ perforations, local irritations due to oxidative processes on the metal surface are rare because only human-tissue-friendly alloys are in use. Small parts, such as clips or needle fragments, are often discovered only by chance. Furthermore, X-ray discovery of retained textiles may be difficult. Despite radio-opaque markings on abdominal sponges, misdiagnoses occur in 3–25% of X-ray, ultrasound, CT, and MRT examinations. The rate of misdiagnoses increases with increasing time elapsed since the initial operation [24]. The reoperation rate is only 70% within two years after surgery, albeit with a considerable mortality rate, between 11–35% [23, 25]. We list the following risk factors for an RSFB event [2]:

- Complex surgical procedures
- Emergency procedures
- Elevated BMI
- Involvement of multiple surgical teams
- Multiple body cavities operated on, e.g., in thoracoabdominal procedures
- Unforeseen intraoperative changes to the surgical procedure
- Need for an unexpectedly large amount of surgical instruments or instrument sets [6, 26–31]

Medical-legal costs associated with RSFBs vary between $37,041 and $2,350,000 even if little harm was done to the patient [2, 32–45]. The average cost of RSFB cases, estimated from three separate studies, was about $95,000 [32, 35, 36].

In a review of over 1,000 cases reported to the National Practitioner Data Bank over a seven-year period, RSFBs are responsible for an average amount of $77,175 paid (maximum payment $2,350,000) in damages as a result of medical malpractice claims [33]. Within the Veterans Health Administration, 103 of 11,066 tort claims, over a 12-year period, were related to RSFBs [2, 34]. An RSFB event is identified as one of 28 "never events" by the National Quality Forum.

If mechanical tackers are used, clips may be lost inside the open abdominal cavity. Usually, they don't cause any problems. In rare cases however, they may cause severe complications, for example, adhesive bands and ensuing ileus [37–41]. For this reason, the surgeon must extract any free intraabdominal clips. If the search for lost clips is not successful, the OR report must at least document the attempt. From opinions issued by the Supreme Court, it may be gathered that in such cases the surgeon is not automatically deemed at fault and that presence of an RSFB does not automatically imply violation of due medical diligence [42, 43]. Juridical assessment depends on the individual case. Retained foreign bodies cannot always be prevented, even if a high degree of diligence was exercised. In a legal context, the decisive factors are type, size, or length of a retained foreign body. Without question, the surgeon is at fault if a large object is left behind, i.e., forceps, scissors, or a large abdominal sponge. In individual cases where small gauze swabs, tamponades, or broken-off needle tips were left behind, culpability was denied. In such cases, the decisive question is whether every reasonably possible precaution was taken to prevent retainment from happening [44].

At this time, no fully reliable method for counting swabs, gauze compresses and needles exists. Counting procedures are even more unreliable if the objects aren't placed on the instrument tray before the beginning of surgery, if an unexpected change to the surgical procedure is necessary, or if unforeseeable intraoperative incidents occur. As mentioned above, counting errors cannot be definitely excluded, which provides a further argument against relying on counting methods. The surgical count itself falls under the responsibility of the medical support staff. Nevertheless, the surgeon is required to question the OR nurse in order to convince himself that sponges, swabs, and instruments have been fully counted. In addition, swabs, surgical strips, and compresses may never be handed to the surgeon separately but must be given in a special clamp with a reliable locking mechanism. Beyond this, the counting procedure must be documented, usually on standardized reply forms with multiple categories, on which pre- and postoperative counting results can be recorded and which are signed by the surgeon after the responsible OR staff has notified him that the count has been completed. If counting is not documented, established jurisprudence in civil law considers it as not carried out at all [43]. In the context of risk management, which each clinic is required to implement, all safety procedures must be regularly reviewed and, if necessary, updated to reflect the latest insights in the field. This includes, e.g., continuous schooling of the OR staff. For example, on the basis of positive results gained from trainings in teamwork, John-Hopkins Hospital (Baltimore) established a system of briefings and debriefings before and after each surgical procedure, thus reducing the risk of errors and improving patient safety [45].

3.3 Risk management related to the prevention of RSFBs

Many hospitals have developed initiatives to reduce the incidence of RSFBs. Innovative techniques, such as radio frequency identification (RFID), can make an important contribution towards this goal.

More basic tools, such as bags for sorting sponges, are already widely used. In order to reduce the incidence of RSFBs, hospitals target imperfections within their own healthcare systems, especially those related to communication deficiencies between members of the surgical team [46, 47]. A national organization has been formed, called "No Thing left Behind", to develop approaches for addressing the RSFB problem and to provide consultancy services to hospitals and healthcare systems [47]. The Association of perioperative Registered Nurses (AORN) maintains the "Safety Net" anonymous reporting tool, which tracks perioperative near-misses. Hospitals can access this data to better understand safety lapses and to consult organizational safety guidelines [48].

In 2009, Stawicki et al. proposed the following summary overview of possible measures to prevent RSFBs:

Tab. 3.1: Measures to prevent retained surgical foreign bodies [2]

- Accurate, repeated, and reproducible counting of surgical instruments and sponges
- Use of automated systems for counting and identifying surgical sponges and instruments
- Detailed exploration of the surgical field prior to wound closure
- Avoiding use of small surgical sponges, avoiding use of sponges or towels that do not contain radio-opaque markers, and simultaneous use of the least number of sponges needed to perform the surgical task at hand

Multiple 'checks and balances' incorporating various RSFB prevention strategies at multiple points during the patient's surgical care
- In the absence of surgical or medical emergency, appropriate safety procedures should never be abandoned or terminated prematurely.
- Establish educational programs aimed at encouraging teamwork and adherence to patient safety protocols.

Radiographs of the anatomic region corresponding to the surgical site must be performed right before or right after fascial closure with the patient still on the operating table
- if intraoperative instrument/sponge counts inconsistent
- during high-risk procedures
- every four days and before definitive abdominal (fascial) closure in staged (damage control) procedures

Use of specialized radio-frequency systems, consisting of a radio-frequency detector and RF-tagged surgical sponges.
- The surgical team must be fully aware of the advantages and limitations of radio-frequency tagging systems, including the fact that certain surgical objects (i.e., instruments, needles, and non-RF-tagged sponges) can not be detected by this method.

Operating room staff consists of human beings, and we may not forget that people can make mistakes. However, organizational, communicative, and educational errors frequently underlie human errors. Individual mistakes often reflect cultural errors, i.e., cultural deficiencies within the hospital.

3.4 Real-life examples

Example 1

A 36-year-old female patient was diagnosed with acute phlegmonous appendicitis, and underwent appendectomy. After an initially inconspicuous postoperative period, the patient developed recurrent abdominal pain for which she was examined by numerous medical specialists over a period of five years. Comprehensive endoscopic diagnostics was conducted, including gastroscopy and colonoscopy, on the basis of which the patient was diagnosed with chronic gastritis, for which she was then treated pharmaceutically for several years. The patient's persisting complaints were attributed to suspected abdominal adhesions. At various times, the patient was treated with antibiotics, due to frequently recurring, unexplained attacks of fever. Eventually, a CT scan showed an artificial, tubular formation in the small intestine. During the ensuing operation, surgeons encountered a conglomerate mass, packed tightly with several intestinal loops. The tissue was removed. Additional extended right side hemicolectomy, sigmoid resection as well as an 85-cm-long jejunal resection were necessary. The dissected tissue was found to contain a retained compress, which had been feeding the longstanding severe inflammatory process.

Example 2

In order to treat pelvic floor descensus, a 70-year-old female patient underwent transvaginal hysterectomy, with augmentation of the pelvic floor. For many months post-op, recurrent blood discharges from the cervical stump were noted. During an ultrasound examination, tumor-like shapes were seen in the abdominal cavity, next to the bladder. An ensuing CT scan showed a garland-like structure with metallic inclusions above the cervical stump. The patient underwent laparotomy, where a purulent, infected swab was removed, which had caused an extended abscess near the cervical stump and in the Douglas space and which had already eroded the bladder wall. During the following lawsuit, the responsible hospital confirmed that no counting procedure had been carried out.

3.5 Summary

Retained surgical foreign objects may remain inside the organism for many years post-op, without causing any symptoms. Even more so, if the object does not cause any infections or allergic reactions such as abscesses, fistulas, perforations, or peritonitis. In other cases, they may be the cause of severe, lasting damage to the patient and a life of suffering. There is an increased risk of RSFBs in emergency situations or if several surgical disciplines need to cooperate in the operating room. To reduce the still unacceptably high number of RSFBs, it is necessary to confront the issue openly and to keep improving risk management strategies.

References

[1] Schönleben, K, Strobel, A, Schönleben, F, Hoffmann, A. Belassene Fremdkörper aus der Sicht des Chirurgen. Chirurg 2007; 78:712.
[2] Stawicki, SP, Evans, DC, Cipolla, J. et al. Retained surgical foreign bodies: A comprehensive review of risks and preventive studies. Scandinavian Journal of Surgery 2009; 98:8–17.
[3] Sarda, AK, Pandey, N, Neogi, S, Dhir, U. Postoperative complications due to a retained surgical sponge. Singapore Med J 2007; 48(6):e160.
[4] Lincourt, AE, Harrell, A, Cristiano, J, Sechris, C. et al. Retained foreign bodies after surgery. Journal of Surgical Research 2007, Volume 138, Issue 2, p. 170–171.
[5] Kaiser, CW, Friedman, S, Spurling, KP. et al. The retained surgical sponge: Ann Surg 1996; 224:79–84. Comment in: Ann Surg 1997; 225:442.

[6] Gawande, AA, Studdert, DM, Orav, EJ, Brennan, TA. et al. Risk factors for retained instruments and sponges after surgery. N Engl J Med 2003; 348:229–235. Comment in: N Engl J Med 2003; 348:1724–5.

[7] Tacyildiz, I, Aldemir, M. The mistakes of surgeons: „gossypiboma". Acta Chir Belg 2004; 104:71–75.

[8] Ribalta, T, McCutcheon, IE, Neto, AG. et al. Textiloma (gossypiboma) mimicking recurrent intracranial tumor. Arch Pathol Lab Med 2004; 128:749–758.

[9] Berger, C, Hartmann, M, Wildemann, B. Progressive visual loss due to a muslinoma – report of a case and review of the literature. Eur J Neurol 2003; 10:153–158.

[10] Mouhsine, E, Halkic, N, Garofalo, R. et al. Soft-tissue textiloma: a potential diagnostic pitfall. Can J Surg 2005; 48:495–496.

[11] Marcy, PY, Hericord, O, Novellas, S. Lymph node-like lesion of the neck after pharyngolaryn-gectomy. AJR Am J Roentgenol 2006; 1878:W135–W136.

[12] Hyslop, JW, Maull, KI. Natural history of the retained surgical sponge. South Med J 1982; 75:657–660.

[13] Imran, Y, Azman, MZ. Asymptomatic chronically retained gauze in the pelvic cavity. Med J Malaysia 2005; 60:358–359.

[14] Gencosmanoglu, R, Inceoglu, R. An unusual cause of small bowel obstruction: gossypiboma – case report. BMC Surg 2003; 3:6.

[15] Bani-Hani, KE, Gharaibeh, KA, Yaghan, RJ. Retained surgical sponges (gossypiboma). Asian J Surg 2005; 28:109–115.

[16] Yildirim, S, Tarim, A, Nursal, TZ. et al. Retained surgical sponge (gossypiboma) after intraab-dominal or retroperitoneal surgery: 14 cases treated at a single centre. Langenbecks Arch Surg 2006; 391(4):390.

[17] Kato, K, Kawai, T, Suzuki, K. et al. Migration of surgical sponge retained at transvaginal hys-terectomy into the bladder: a case report. Hinyokika Klyo 1998; 44(3):183.

[18] Apter, S, Hertz, M, Rubinstein, ZJ, Zissin, R. Gossypiboma in the early post-operative period: a diagnostic problem. Clin Radiol 1990; 42(2):128.

[19] Klein, J, Farman, J, Burrell, M. et al. The forgotten surgical foreign body. Gastrointest Radiol 1988; 13(2):173.

[20] Mason, LB. Migration of surgical sponge into small intestine. JAMA 1968; 205(13):938.

[21] Rappaport, W, Haynes, K. The retained surgical sponge following intra-abdominal surgery. A continuing problem. Arch Surg 1990; 125(3):405.

[22] Risher, WH, McKinnon, WM. Foreign body in the gastrointestinal tract: intraluminal migra-tion of laparotomy sponge. South Med J 1991; 84(8):1042.

[23] Wig, JD, Goenka, MK, Suri, S. et al. Retained surgical sponge: an unusual cause of intestinal obstruction. J Clin Gastroenterol 1991; 24(1):57.

[24] Revesz, G, Siddiqi, TS, Buchheit, WA, Bonitatibus, M. Detection of retained surgical sponges. Radiology 1983; 149(2):411.

[25] Lauwers, PR, van Hee, RH. Intraperitoneal gossypibomas: the need of count sponges. World J Surg 2000; 24(5):521.

[26] Teixeira, PG, Inaba, K, Salim, A. et al. Retained foreign bodies after emergent trauma surgery: incidence after 2526 cavitary explorations. Am Surg 2007; 73:1031–1034.

[27] Imren, Y, Rasoglu, I, Ozkose, Z. A different intracardiac mass: retained sponge. Echocardio-graphy 2006; 23:322–323.

[28] Hadrami, J, Rojas, M, de Fenoyl, O. et al. Pulmonary texiloma revealed by haemoptysis 12 years after thoracotomy. Rev Med Interne 1998; 19:826–829.

[29] Roumen, RM, Weerdenburg, HP. MR features of a 24-year-old gossypiboma. A case report. Acta Radiol 1998; 39:176–178.

[30] Egorova, NN, Moskowitz, A, Gelijns, A. et al. Managing the prevention of retained surgical instruments: what is the value of counting? Ann Surg 2008; 247:13–18.

[31] Stawicki, SP, Cipolla, J, Bria, C. Comparison of open abdomens in non-trauma and trauma patients: a retrospective study: OPUS 12 Scientist 2007; 1(1):1–8.

[32] Berkowitz, S, Marshall, H, Charles, A. Retained intra-abdominal surgical instruments: time to use nascent technology? Am Surg 2007; 73:1083–1085.

[33] National Practitioner Data Bank Public Data file: Available online at: www.npdb-hipdb.hrsa. gov/pubs/stats/Public_Use_Data:_File.pdf. Last accessed on July 28, 2008.

[34] Weeks, WB, Foster, T, Wallace, AE. et al. Tort Claims Analysis in the Veteran Health Administration for Quality Improvement. The Journal of Law. Medicine & Ethics 2001; 29:335–345.

[35] Smith, C. Surgical tools left in five patients. Available online at: http://seattlepi.nwsource.com/local/49883_error08.shtml. Last accessed on March 12, 2008.

[36] Dippolito, A, Braslow, BM, Lombardo, G. et al. How David beat Goliath: history of physicians fighting frivolous law suits. OPUS 12 Scientist 2008; 2(1):1–8.

[37] Ashton, P, Kuhn, R, Collopy, B. Small bowel incarceration after laparoscopically assisted vaginal hysterectomy – a preventable complication? Aust N Z J Obstet Gynaecol 1995; 35:352.

[38] Huntington, TR, Klomp, GR. Retained staples as a cause of mechanical small bowel obstruction. Surg Endosc 1995; 9:353.

[39] Jenkins, DM, Paluzzi, M, Scott, TE. Postlaparoscopic small bowel obstruction. Surg Laparosc Endos 1993; 3:139.

[40] Sauer, M, Jarrett, JC. Small bowel obstruction following diagnostic laparoscopy. Fertil Steril 1984; 42:653.

[41] Lörken, M, Marnitz, U, Schumpelick, V. Freier intraperitonealer Clip als Ursache eines mechanischen Dünndarmileus. Chirurg 1999; 70:1492–1493.

[42] BGH, VersR 1953, 338; VersR 1964, 392; VersR 1955, 344.

[43] Ulsenheimer, K. Belassene Fremdkörper aus der Sicht des Juristen. Chirurg 2007; 78:28–34.

[44] BGH, Urteil v. 27.11.1981 – VIZR 138/79.

[45] Makary, MA, Sexton, JB, Freischlag, JA. et al. Patient safety in surgery. Ann Surg 2006; 243(5):628.

[46] Aleccia, J. MSNBC Health Care. Medical litter: device debris poses serious risk. Available online at: http://msnbc.msn.com/id/25120613/. Last accessed on July 28, 2008.

[47] Frangou, C. Mayo study counts surgical objects left behind. General Surgery News 2008; 35:18–19.

[48] Beyea, S. Counting instruments and sponges. AORN J 2003; 78:290–292.

4 Quality management related to wrong-site surgery

4.1 Introduction

Mix-ups of surgical procedures or patients are unacceptable and may have fatal consequences. Zero-tolerance error management is the only answer to the still large number of mix-ups. Numerous international initiatives have been started that try to sustainably reduce the number of mix-ups to, ideally, zero.

4.2 Statistical surveys

The consequences of adverse events involving wrong-side/wrong-site, wrong-procedure, and wrong-patient errors (WSPEs) are devastating and unacceptable. A WSPE can be defined as any procedure that has been performed on the opposite side, at an incorrect site or at the wrong level, or on the wrong patient, and includes cases where the wrong procedure was performed. Wrong-procedure and wrong-patient errors may have different causes, but they often share underlying basic error pathology related to ambiguous and imprecise identification [1] which is often rooted in communication breakdown or lack of safety systems to prevent these types of errors [2]. It is possible, that the peculiarities of the human neurological and cognitive equipment predispose to such mix-ups [3]. In the English-speaking world, the various types of mix-ups are often summarized under the heading of "wrong-site surgery". The frequency with which mix-ups occur is most certainly underestimated and the medical literature on the topic is both scarce and limited in scope. On the other hand, the topic has repeatedly been discussed at conferences, based on individual case studies. Kwaan et al. evaluated wrong-site surgeries reported to a large medical malpractice insurer between 1985 and 2004. Based on the reported claims and excluding spinal surgery, they determined an incidence of only one in 112,994 procedures [4].

To put it another way, at any one hospital, wrong-site surgery was reported to insurance companies and/or caused a lawsuit once every five years [4]. From 1985 to 1995, the Physicians' Insurance Association of America reviewed claims data from 22 malpractice carriers, insuring a total number of 110,000 physicians [5]. The study revealed that wrong-site surgery occurred in 331 cases and was responsible for 1,000 closed malpractice suits. During their first year of public reporting, the state of Minnesota reported 26 wrong-site surgeries. During their second year, 31 cases were reported [6, 7]. In Virginia, wrong-site surgery was reported for one out of 30,000 surgeries, which is about one incident per month [8]. In the State of New York, over the year 2001, wrong-site surgery was reported for one in 15,500 surgeries [8].

A few Swedish cases were reported as early as the 1970s [9–12]. Seiden et al. [1] collected further, sporadic case reports. In the period 1995–2006, 532 reports involving sentinel events caused by wrong-site surgery were referred to the Joint Commission on Accreditation of Healthcare Organizations (JCAHO) [13]. During a 35-year career, an orthopedic surgeon has a 25% risk of performing a wrong-side operation [14]. In hand surgery, the incidence of left/right mix-ups is estimated at once per 27,686 procedures [15]. Cowell [16] reported 331 cases of wrong-site surgery over a 16-year period. These, however, are all based on self-reports or surveys and almost certainly underestimate the real incidence of WSPEs, possibly by a factor of 20 or more [15, 17, 18]. Seiden et al. [1] reviewed WSPE data collected from 4 databases:

1. The National Practitioner Data Bank (NPDB);
2. the Florida Code 15 mandatory reporting system;
3. the American Society of Anaesthesiologists (ASA) Closed Claims Project database;
4. the ASA's novel WSPE incident reporting tool.

Out of 236,300 cases, the National Practitioner Data Bank (NPDP) contained 2,217 cases (0.94%) designated "wrong-body-part surgery" and 3,723 cases designated "wrong-treatment/wrong-procedure performed". The annual frequencies of WSPE incidents recorded in the NPDB, ranged from 359 to 457 cases over the period 1998–1999.

Since 1991, 494 well-documented WSPE incidents have been reported to the state of Florida, with an average 75 events per year since 2000 [19]. In this report, radiological mistakes took first place, with second place taken by cataract surgery and third place by inguinal hernia surgery. Based on this data, the total amount of left/right mix-ups in the USA is estimated at 1,321 cases per year [20]. Hence, wrong-side events turn out to be much more frequent than was generally assumed or at least than has been published in the literature. With 1,300 to 2,700 cases in more than 75 million operations per year, the incidence of WSPEs in the USA is more than 5–10 times larger than the manufacturing industry's quality-defect standard, the so-called six sigma norm [21]. Wrong-implant surgery has occurred in obstetrics (wrong-embryo implantation) [22–24] and in eye surgery (wrong lenses implanted or surgery on the wrong side) [28]. Several publications report mix-ups where, e.g., the wrong knee or finger was operated [26, 27]. Patient mix-ups may have dramatic consequences. For example, the German layman press reported the case of a 76-year-old woman, who was to be operated on her knee. Due to a mistaken diagnosis with rectal carcinoma, abdominoperineal rectal extirpation was performed and the patient woke up from anesthesia with an artificial stoma [25]. In cancer surgery, the consequences may be outright catastrophic, if, e.g., the wrong breast is amputated or the wrong half of the lungs resected. There have even been reports of mistaken identity in cases where life support was withdrawn [29], radiation therapy was given [30], or tonsillectomy was performed [31]. Another case involved an ABO-incompatible heart-lung transplantation due to mistaken identity [32]. The consequences of such mix-ups range from a prolonged stay in hospital to patient death and may be devastating for surgeon, OR team, and hospital alike.

4.3 Root cause analysis

A zero-tolerance policy is the only standard that can be ethically justified by care providers and will be accepted by patients and the general public alike. Preventive mechanisms require specific attention to organizational and cultural barriers that affect patient safety strategies. One of the greatest barriers to the elimination of WSPEs is that, paradoxically, they occur relatively infrequently, and health care providers usually believe themselves immune to such human errors [1]. Healthcare systems in both the USA and Europe do not have a sufficient nationwide culture of organizational structuring at their disposal, which might effectively prevent this class of mistakes. WSPEs are caused by multiple systemic and organizational factors, including similarity of surgical sites, similar names of patients and surgical procedures, breakdowns in communication and teamwork, procedural and patient-related factors, and failure of those safety checks that are already in place.

Tab. 4.1: Factors contributing to WSPEs, determined from case analyses [1]

Human factors
- High workload environment
- Fatigue
- Multiple team members involved
- Diffusion of authority/lack of accountability
- Team communication
- Change of personnel
- Haste
- Inexperience
- Incompetence
- Other cognitive factors

Patient-related factors
- Sedation or anesthesia
- Patient not consulted before block or anesthesia
- Patient confusion of side, site, or procedure
- Inability to engage patient (e.g., young children or decreased competence)
- Patient ignorance
- Patient has common name or same name as another patient in hospital

Procedural factors
- Wrong side draped/prepped
- Similar or same procedures back to back in same operating room
- Patient position or room changed prior to initiating procedure
- Attempts to prevent WSPE
- Not observing marked site/marking wrong site
- Failure to cross-check for consistency of consent form, patient chart, and/or booking room

An examination of 27,370 consecutive adverse events, reported to the Colorado Physician Insurance Company (COPIC) during the study period from January 1, 2002 to June 1, 2008, revealed 119 cases of wrong-site surgery and 29 cases of wrong-patient surgery, distributed over the various surgical specialisms as outlined in the following table:

Tab. 4.2: Overview of physicians involved in wrong-patient or wrong-site surgeries [33]

	No. (%)	
Characteristics	**Wrong Patient (n = 25)**	**Wrong Site (n = 107)**
Nonsurgical specialisms		
Dermatology, nonprocedural	1 (4.0)	4 (3.7)
Emergency medicine	0	2 (1.9)
Family or general practice	2 (8.0)	4 (3.7)
Internal medicine	6 (24.0)	8 (7.5)
Neurology	0	1 (0.9)
Ophthalmology, nonprocedural	0	1 (0.9)
Pathology	2 (8.0)	1 (0.9)
Pediatrics	2 (8.0)	1 (0.9)
Radiation oncology	0	3 (2.8)
Radiology	1 (4.0)	4 (3.7)
Surgical		
Anesthesiology	0	13 (12.1)
Dermatology, procedural	0	2 (1.9)
Otorhinolaryngology	1 (4.0)	1 (0.9)
General surgery	0	18 (16.8)
Obstetrics-gynecology	2 (8.0)	1 (0.9)
Ophthalmology, procedural	0	1 (0.9)
Orthopedic surgery	0	24 (22.4)
Neurosurgery	0	2 (1.9)
Urology	2 (8.0)	4 (3.7)
Other	6 (24.0)	12 (11.2)
Sex		
Female	6 (24.0)	14 (13.1)
Male	11 (44.0)	80 (74.8)
Unknown	8 (32.0)	13 (12.1)
Practice type		
Ambulatory surgery center	2 (8.0)	24 (22.4)
Hospital	8 (32.0)	62 (57.9)
Office	9 (36.0)	13 (12.1)
Nursing home	1 (4.0)	0
Other	5 (20.0)	8 (7.5)

The specialisms most frequently involved in wrong-site incidents were orthopedic surgery (22.4%), general surgery (16.8%), and anesthesiology (12.1%). This study documented a high incidence of surgical never events, with 25 cases of wrong-patient surgery and 107 wrong-site surgeries.

Root cause analysis reveals a high incidence of diagnostic errors, which result in wrong-patient procedures in more than half of all cases (56%). These incidents could have been avoided by formally implementing preoperative patient re-identification. Communication errors were identified as contributing root causes in all wrong-patient incidents [33]. This data agrees with other studies, which also identified communication breakdown as a leading cause of wrong-site surgery [34]. A root cause analysis of wrong-procedure incidents during electrophysiological procedures, by Chassin and Becher [35], showed 17 different mistakes, none of which had single-handedly caused the sentinel event. Rather, it was the combination of several mistakes which had caused the incident.

In August 1998, the Joint Commission issued a Sentinel Event Alert, examining the problem of wrong-site surgery, which included a review of 15 cases reported to the JCAHO.

The Joint Commission identified a number of factors contributing to an increased risk of wrong-site, wrong-person, or wrong-procedure surgery, including:

- More than one surgeon was involved in the case, because either multiple procedures were contemplated or the patient was handed over to another surgeon.
- Multiple procedures were conducted on the same patient during a single operation. This was especially significant if it involved different sides of the patient.
- There was an unusual time pressure due to an unusual starting time or pressure to speed up preoperative procedures.
- There were unusual patient characteristics in play, such as physical deformity or massive obesity, which may alter usual equipment set-up or patient-positioning procedures.

Communication breakdowns can be divided into two categories:

- Failure to engage the patient (or family) in the process of identifying the correct surgical site, either during the informed consent procedure or by asking him to mark the intended surgical site.
- Incomplete or inaccurate communication between members of the surgical team, often due to the exclusion of OR team members from participating in the site verification process or through single reliance on the surgeon's determination of the site. In many cases, procedures to verify the surgical site were found to be flawed, for example, due to the following factors:
  — deviations from normal procedures
  — absence of re-verification of the surgical site in the operating room
  — absence of verbal communication between team members during site verification
  — not all relevant information available in the operation room
  — no checklist to ensure that all relevant steps of the verification process were taken
  — team members not feeling permitted to point out possible errors
  — sole reliance on the surgeon for verifying the surgical site, after the adage: "the surgeon should never be questioned"

4.4 Risk management related to the prevention of WSPEs

On July 1, 2004, the Joint Commission on Accreditation of Health Care Organizations (JCAHO) implemented the universal protocol for the prevention of WSPEs [36].

This Universal Protocol consists of three steps outlined in Table 4.3.

Tab. 4.3: Universal Protocol of the Joint Commission on Accreditation of Health Care Organizations (JCAHO)

1. **Preoperative verification to ensure that all relevant documents and studies are complete and available.**

    - Ensure that all relevant documents and studies are available prior to the start of the procedure and that they have been reviewed and are consistent with each other, with the patient's expectations, and with the team's understanding of the intended patient, procedure, site, and, if applicable, any implants. Missing information or discrepancies must be addressed before staring the procedure.
    - This verification includes:
        — patient identification with at least two identifiers (e.g., patient name, medical record number, date of birth)
        — medical history and results from physical examinations, documented in the patient's records
        — signed consent form in the medical record, with verification of the procedure
        — mark and verify the surgical site, if possible, with involvement of the patient. This is mandatory for procedures involving right/left distinction, multiple structures, e.g., fingers, toes, or multiple levels in spinal operations. The site must be marked with "YES", such that the mark will be visible after the patient has been prepared for surgery and is lying on the operating table. In most cases, the physician performing the procedure will be responsible for marking the site.
    - Process: an ongoing process of information gathering and verification, that begins with the decision for surgical intervention and continues through all settings and interventions involved in the preoperative preparation of the patient, up to and including the "time out" just before the start of the operation.

2. **Preoperative marking of the surgical site.**

    - Process: For procedures involving left/right distinction, multiple structures, such as fingers and toes, or multiple levels in spinal procedures, the intended site must be marked such that the mark will be visible after the patient has been prepped and draped.

    The site must be marked with a "Yes", so that the mark will be visible. In most cases, the physician performing the procedure is responsible for marking the site.

3. **Time Out (final verification).**

    The Time Out is a deliberate pause to allow for clear communication between all members of the surgical team (including active listening and verbal confirmation of patient, procedure, site, and side). The procedure is not started until all questions or concerns are resolved. The Time Out includes verifying:

    - Patient identity
    - Patient informed consent
    - Surgical site and side (verified with site marking as per policy)
    - Position of the patient on the operating table
    - Availability of correct implants and any special equipment or other required items

When developing this protocol, consensus was reached on the following principles:

- Wrong-site, wrong-procedure, and wrong-person surgery must be prevented.
- A robust approach, using multiple, complementary strategies, is necessary to achieve the goal of eliminating wrong-site, wrong-procedure, and wrong-person surgery.
- Active involvement of and effective communication between all members of the surgical team is important to a successful outcome.
- The patient (or legally designated representative) should be involved in the process to the maximum extent possible.
- Consistent implementation of a standardized approach, using a universal, consensus-based protocol will be most effective.
- The protocol should be flexible enough to allow for implementing appropriate adaptations if required to meet the specific needs of individual patients.
- The requirement to mark the surgical site should focus on cases involving right/left distinction, multiple structures (fingers, toes), or levels (spine).
- The universal protocol should be applicable or adaptable to all operative and other invasive procedures that expose patients to harm, including procedures that are performed in settings other than the operating room.

However, the analysis by Stahel et al. [33] showed that implementation of the universal protocol has not yet led to a lower incidence of WSPEs.

Surgical never events also occur in nonsurgical areas, which means that the Universal Protocol must not be limited to the classic procedural or operative disciplines but must be universally implemented [33]. The World Health Organization's Patient Safety Program "Safe Surgery Saves Lives" has developed a surgical safety checklist as a means of improving worldwide safety of surgical care. A multinational study involving eight hospitals from diverse economical settings showed that the use of this checklist improved compliance with standards of care by 65% and reduced the mortality rate after surgery by nearly 50% [37]. In the current era of the Universal Protocol, inadequate planning and lack of adherence to the Time Out principle seem to be the major determinants of adverse outcome. Stahel demanded strict adherence to the Universal Protocol and an increase of its scope to include the non-surgical disciplines.

This WHO-developed checklist "Safe Surgery Saves Life" consists of three phases:

1. Sign-In: patient identification, informed consent, and verification of safety-relevant patient data, e.g., anticoagulant medication, allergies, prior issues with regard to anesthesia, and expected intraoperative blood loss.
2. Time-Out: each team member introduces himself by stating name and role in the team. Verification of patient, disease, and planned operation. Review of medical imaging results and of critical steps in the procedure.
3. Sign-Out: renewed review of the operation. Counting the number of instruments, compresses, abdominal swabs, etc. and review of postoperative management.

The German Alliance for Patient Safety has developed a standardized form to help prevent wrong-procedure events, which by now has been implemented in many clinics. It consists of four steps:

1. Informed consent, ascertained by a fully informed physician or surgeon. The patient's identity is verified. The procedure is reviewed and the surgical site

determined together with the patient. Under circumstances, the patient's relatives (for children) must be included to the extent possible.

2. For procedures involving left/right distinction, the surgical site is marked by the surgeon or fully informed physician, with a waterproof felt-tip pen, outside of the operating room, with the patient not yet under medication. The patient must actively contribute to the process by pointing out and verifying the site.

3. After transferal to the surgical area, the OR staff verifies the patient's identity by asking him to state his name and date of birth. Before the patient enters the operating room proper, the anesthesiologist verifies the patient's identity as well as the location and proper marking of the surgical site. If any discrepancies exist, the surgeon must be consulted prior to induction of anesthesia.

4. Time-Out, immediately prior to surgery. The accompanying documentation sheet is added to the patient's records. Acceptance of the "Time-Out" by all of the staff can be ensured only if surgeons and head physicians set the example by its habitual implementation. This procedure is accepted and deemed exemplary also by the Joint Commission in the USA [38, 39].

Nevertheless, the implementation of the above procedure must be regularly monitored. At the moment, only 75% of the total number of standardized forms is filled out [40].

Clearly, despite the various protocols mentioned, left/right mix-ups cannot be prevented in all cases. Seiden et al. reported several cases of wrong-side events due to the patient being mistaken, despite being awake and fully conscious. These patients, one of whom was himself a surgeon, would not have been capable of pointing out the mistake to the OR team and halt the erroneous operation. From one of these patients, the only still-functioning kidney was removed. Another patient, suffering from aphasia after a stroke, underwent bilateral orchiectomy instead of circumcision [1, 40, 41].

In addition, adherence to the guideline that demands patient participation has been low. DiGiovanni et al. [42] found low compliance rates for patients marking their operative site. Out of 100 patients included in the study, 59% correctly marked the surgical site, 37% did not mark it, and 4% did not mark it correctly.

Recent data suggests that one third of wrong-site incidents occurred in spite of careful implementation of identification procedures, similar to the JCAHO universal protocol [4]. Although comprehensive data is lacking, WSPEs have been shown to occur even after implementation of the universal protocol [43]. Hence, procedures for reporting and responding to wrong-site surgery or near misses are necessary. These procedures are key points in any WSPE policy and constitute important steps in reducing their incidence [44]. Kwaan et al. [4] obtained 16 such protocols and found that in at least one third of the analyzed wrong-site surgery cases, they would not have prevented the incident.

4.5 Summary

Because of differences of opinion and fear of litigation, it is unlikely that WSPEs will always be fully reported. Many healthcare organizations, drawing on theories of error prevention and experience gained from the aviation industry, recognize that transparency in dealing with these problems may induce changes to the system, resulting in a better outcome for the patient.

References

[1] Seiden, SC, Barach, P. Wrong-side/wrong-site, wrong-procedure, and wrong-patient adverse events. Archives of Surgery, 2006; vol 141, No 9:931–939.

[2] Reason, JT. Managing the Risks of Organizational Accidents: Aldershot, Hants, England. Brookfield, Vt. Ashgate, 1997.

[3] Storfer, M.D. Problems in left-right discrimination in a high-IQ population. Perception Mot Skills. 1995; 81:491–497.

[4] Kwaan, MR, Studdert, DM, Zinner, M.J. Incidence, patterns, and prevention of wrong-site surgery. Arch Surg 2006; 141:353–357.

[5] Shojania, KG, Duncan, BW, McDonald, KM. et al. eds. Making Healthcare Safer: A Critical Analysis of Patient Safety Practices. Subchapter 43.2. Strategies to avoid wrong-site surgery. Evidence Report/Technology Assessment No. 43, AHRQ Publication No. 01-E058. Rockville. MD: Agency for Healthcare Research and Quality; 2001; 498–503.

[6] Minnesota Department of Health. Adverse health events in Minnesota: second annual public report. [Minnesota Department for Health Web site]. February 2006: Available at www.health.state.mn.us/patientsafety/ae/aereport0206.pdf. Accessed April 24, 2007.

[7] Minnesota Department of Health. Adverse health events in Minnesota: third annual public report. [Minnesota Department for Health Web site]. January 2007: Available at www.health.state.mn.us/patientsafety/ae/aereport0107.pdf. Accessed April 24, 2007.

[8] Dunn, D. Surgical site verification: A through Z. J Perianesth Nurs. 2006; 21:317–331.

[9] Kidney puncture on the wrong-side caution [in Swedish]. Lakartidningen. 1975; 72:793.

[10] Ureter surgery of the wrong side [in Swedish]. Tidskr Sver Sjukskot. 1975; 42:62.

[11] Femur operation on the wrong side [in Swedish]. Lakartidningen. 1976; 73:1327.

[12] Hip surgery on the wrong-side [in Swedish]. Vardfacket. 1977; 1:68.

[13] Joint Commission. Sentinel event statistics. 2007. http://www.jointcommission.org/NR/. Accessed April 24, 2007.

[14] Canale, ST. Wrong-site surgery: a preventable complication. Clin Orthop Relat Res 2005; 433:26–29.

[15] Meinberg, EG, Stern, PJ. Incidence of wrong-site surgery among hand surgeons. J Bone Joint Surg [Am] 2003; 85:193–197.

[16] Cowell, HR. Wrong-site surgery [editorial]. J Bone Joint Surg Am. 1998; 80:463.

[17] Barach, P, Small, SD. Reporting and preventing medical mishaps: lessons from non-medical near miss reporting systems. BMJ 2000; 320:759–763.

[18] Bates, DW, Cullen, DJ, Laird, N. et al. ADE Prevention Study Group. Incidence of adverse drug events and potential adverse drug events: Implications for prevention. JAMA. 1995; 274:29–34.

[19] AHCA. Florida Agency for Healthcare Administration Web site. 2003. http://www.fdhc.state.fl.us/. Accessed June 18, 2006.

[20] Ranking tables for states: population in 2000 and population change from 1990 to 2000 (PHC-T-2). US Census Bureau Web site. Revised July 31, 2002. http://www.census.gov/population/www/cen2000/phc-t2.html. Accessed June 16, 2006.

[21] FAQs. What is Six Sigma? Motorola University, Motorola Inc Web site. http://www.motorola.com/content.jsp?globalObjectId=3088. Accessed on June 14, 2006.

[22] Chlang, H. Mom awarded $ 1 million over embryo mix-up. San Francisco Chronicle. August 4, 2004; B4. http://sfgate.com/cgi-bin/article.cgi?file=/chronicle/archive/2004/08/04/BAGN382BII1.DTL. Accessed November 28, 2005.

[23] Seligman, K. License revoked for embryo mix-up. San Francisco Chronicle. March 31, 2005; B.4. http://sfgate.com/cgi-bin/article.cgi?file=/c/a/2005/03/31/BAGIOC10PK1.DTL. Accessed November 28, 2005.

[24] Wright, O. Wrong embryos implanted in three patients. The Times (London). October 29, 2002; Home news: 4.

[25] American Academy of Ophthalmology. Minimizing wrong IOL placement: patient safety bulletin number 2. AAO Web site. http://www.aao.org/aao/education/library/safety/iol.cfm. Accessed November 28, 2005.

[26] Joint Commission on Accreditation of Healthcare Organizations. Sentinel event statistics. December 31, 2005. JCAHO Web site. http://www.jointcommission.org/SentinelEvents/Statistics/. Accessed June 24, 2006.

[27] Furey, A, Stone, C, Martin, R. Preoperative signing of the incision site in orthopedic surgery in Canada: J Bone Joint Surg Am. 2002; 84-A:1066–1068.

[28] Imhof, M. Behandlungsfehler in der Medizin. Was nun? Schulz-Kirchner-Verlag 2010.

[29] Associated Press. Hospital pulls plug on the wrong patient. Toronto Star. March 13, 1995; A.2.

[30] Radiation given to wrong patient. The Gazette. December 2, 1992; Section A:3.

[31] Mishra, R. Wrong girl gets tonsils taken out. Boston Globe. December 23, 2000; Section B:1.

[32] Archibold, RC. Girl in transplant mix-up dies after two weeks. New York Times. February 23, 2003; 1:18.

[33] Stahel, PhF, Sabel, AL, Victoroff, MS. et al. Wrong-site and wrong-patient procedures in the Universal Protocol Era. Arch Surg 2010; 145(10):978–984.

[34] Makary, MA, Mukherjee, A, Sexton, JB. et al. Operating room briefings and wrong-site surgery. J Am Coll Surg. 2007; 204(2):236–243.

[35] Chassin, MR, Becher, EC. The wrong patient. Ann Int Med 2002; 136:826–833.

[36] Joint Commission on Accreditation of Healthcare Organizations. Guidelines for implementing the universal protocol for preventing wrong site, wrong procedure, wrong person surgery. JCAHO Web site. http://www.jointcommission.org/standards_information/up.aspx. Accessed July 7, 2012.

[37] Harrington, JW. Surgical time outs in a combat zone. AORN J. 2009; 89(3):535–537.

[38] Weiser, ThG, Haynes, AB, Lashoher, A. et al. Perspectives in quality: designing the WHO Surgical Safety checklist. International Journal for Quality in Health Care. 2010; Vol 22, No 5.

[39] Haynes, AB, Weiser, TG, Berry, WR. et al. A surgical safety checklist to reduce morbidity and mortality in a global population. N Engl J Med 2009; 360:491–499.

[40] Reuter, F. Vermeidung von Eingriffsverwechslungen. Unfallchirurg 2009, 112:675–678.

[41] Strelec, SR. Anaesthesia and surgery: not always a one-sided affair. ASA Newsletter. http://www.asahg.org/Newsletters/1996/06_96/feature4.htm. Accessed November 28, 2005.

[42] Di Giovanni, CW, Kang, L, Manuel, J. Patient compliance in avoiding wrong-site surgery. J Bone Joint Surg Am. 2003; 85-A:815–819.

[43] O'Leary, DS, Jacott, WE. Mark my limb. AHRQ Morbidity & Mortality Rounds on the Web. December 2004. http://webmm.ahrq.gov/case.aspx?caseID=82. Accessed August 28, 2005.

[44] Patient safety first alert – implementing a correct site surgery policy and procedure. AORN J 2002; 76:785–788.

5 Towards a preventive safety culture within the hospital

5.1 Introduction

In systems as complex as modern medicine, individual and team errors cannot be prevented. Organizational structures in modern hospitals are characterized by a highly differentiated division of labor and by complex interactions between multiple specialisms and occupational categories. Deficient information exchange at these interfaces is a major cause of errors and violations of various degrees of severity. The analysis of mistakes and the modeling of error development, together with implementation of the results from these processes in everyday clinical practice, are the foundations of preventive error management. Fault-tolerant systems must be developed that are in and of themselves capable of compensating for errors or malfunctions, and structures must be created within which competent error handling is required from all staff members on all organizational levels.

5.2 Safety culture

There exist numerous approaches to developing models and concepts for establishing the idea of a safety culture. "Culture is arguably the most elusive term in the generally rather fluid vocabulary of the social sciences" [1]. The British "Health and Safety Commission" has defined the concept of safety culture as being part of organizational culture. This definition comprises the product of individual and collective values, attitudes, perceptions, skills, and behavioral patterns that determine both nature and extent of an organization's internal error handling [2]. According to J.T. Reason, more than 100 million errors are made in cockpits of commercial airliners every year. However, in only 100 cases they result in larger incidents [3, 4]. In the industry, it has been known for decades that, when dealing with complex systems, it is impossible to exclude all risks of error. However, in the capital goods manufacturing industry, any ex post revision of manufacturing defects comes at a high cost. Hence, the economical point of view alone requires establishing safety culture within the context of comprehensive risk and quality management. Numerous methods and instruments from the field of risk and quality management are used to implement safety culture within an organization. As examples, we offer the concept of Total Quality Management (TQM), introduced by Deming and others [5, 6], the zero-defects concept, developed in 1961 by Crosby [7], and importantly also the Six Sigma ($6\,\sigma$) quality management strategy, developed in the USA by Motorola and General Electrics [8–10]. The worldwide effort to analyze all errors and mistakes has led to crucial improvements in aviation safety. In the year 2009, according to the International Aviation Transport Association (IATA), the number of accidents has decreased by a further 36%. Whereas in 2000, one accident happened every 900,000 flights, only 1.2 accidents per 1.2 million flights were registered in 2009.

The above methods aim at continuous process optimization, so that the specified targets may be reached. In these optimization processes, the DMAIC cycle (define-measure-analyze-improve-control) plays a central role.

When the six sigma level has been achieved, only 3.4 defects per million opportunities may be expected. However, this level is not acceptable for high security sectors such as civil aviation and the offshore and nuclear industries, which require zero-tolerance policies [11]. According to Park [12], the probability of human error increases with the amount of people involved and the number of separate steps in the operating procedure.

The first steps in the scientific treatment of the analysis of errors and their origins dates back to the early 20th century when, e.g., Keenan et al. [13] studied accident probabilities in automobile factories. It was the 1986 Chernobyl disaster in particular, [14–17] that triggered a rapid and dynamic acceleration of comprehensive scientific elaborations on the concept of "safety culture". However, other major accidents, such as the London King's Cross subway station fire in 1987 or the explosion of the oil rig "Piper Alpha" in 1988 [18, 19], also contributed to this.

Any safety culture postulates the inherent fallibility of any human being and hence, by looking at it from a systemic perspective, accepts the necessity of learning lessons from any errors that occur [20]. With this, we come back full circle to the subject of medicine. Every patient knows that a zero error rate during treatment is highly unlikely but, being directly affected, his personal expectation will correspond to at least the six sigma level. Over the past few decades, based on the above observations, the medical world has been increasingly dealing with the issue by trying to exploit the experiences gained in high-risk industry sectors and in civil aviation in order to establish safety culture within the framework of medical quality management [21, 22]. After the publication of "To err is human" [23], a rapidly increasing number of publications appeared worldwide, discussing cases of medical malpractice and other errors in patient treatment, occurring in hospitals and within the healthcare system as a whole. This was accompanied by an increasing number of reports on the issue from both government and specialists, calling for improvements in patient safety [24–28]. As early as 1960–1961, Schimmel [29] phrased the difficulties in balancing benefits against possible damage when evaluating measures to improve patient safety as follows:

"… Modern medicine, however, has introduced procedures that cannot always be used harmlessly. To seek absolute safety is to advocate therapeutic nihilism. The dangers of new measures must be accepted as generally warranted by their benefits and should not preclude their useful employment. Until safer procedures evolve however, physicians will best serve their patients by weighing each measure according to its goals and risks, by choosing only those that have been justified, and by remaining prepared to alter the procedures when imminent or actual harm threatens to obliterate their good".

5.3 Error management as part of quality management in the hospital

As a component of quality management, error management is characterized by clearly defined measures, which are operationalized to the extent possible and implemented within an existing organizational structure. These measures target minimization of error rate and maximization of patient safety based on safety culture as the sum of all measures taken to record, analyze, remedy, and prevent errors on all organizational levels. Its first target is to establish safety awareness in the first place. According to the British "Health and Safety Commission", safety culture comprises the product of individual and collective values, attitudes, perceptions, skills, and behavioral patterns that determine the scope, nature and extent of an organization's internal error handling, that is, within the hospital) [2]. Hence, safety culture is a subsystem of the higher-level organizational climate, is influenced by it and is embedded within its framework of values. This cultural background is decisive for the way errors are interpreted - either as obnoxious incidents or as a chance for change and improvement. Hence, in this context, authors such as Rybowiak et al. [19, 30] prefer speaking of "error orientation".

Handling of errors and risks does not consist of analysis of past mistakes alone but targets the question of how to treat and prevent (potential) future errors. We must discriminate between person-oriented and systemic or integrative error analysis models. The aim is to analyze actual errors, potential errors, and risk factors. The results of these analyses are fed back into the elements that constitute an organization's safety culture.

The "error orientation questionnaire" (EOQ), a survey tool designed by Rybowiak et al. [30] to measure error orientation, features the following eight factors:

1. error competence
2. learning from error
3. error risk-taking
4. error strain
5. error anticipation
6. covering up errors
7. error communication
8. thinking about errors

Baer et al. [19, 31] reviewed the positive influence of an organization's error management culture on its performance as a company and concluded that an organization's safety culture cannot be modeled by sole aggregation of individual employees' stances on error management.

The safety culture analysis model after Schüttelkopf (2008) [32] provides a further approach to operationalizing safety culture. In this approach, safety culture rests on three central internal organizational pillars: norms and values, skills, and in-house equipment.

According to J.T. Reason, any well-functioning safety culture rests on the development of effective safety information systems. His conception assumes four cultural components, which sum up to constitute an organization's safety and information culture:

1. reporting culture
2. just culture
3. flexible culture
4. learning culture.

The first of these four central requirements involves the design of reporting systems in conjunction with organization-wide registration and analysis of incidents and near-misses. In order for this system to provide an effective analysis of errors and accidents, all participants must possess an approximately equal amount of information or at least be able to retrieve all relevant information in some standardized form [33].

J.T. Reason oriented himself to reporting systems that have been successfully employed in the aviation industry, such as NASA's "Aviation Safety Reporting System" (ASRS) and the "British Airways Safety Information System" (BASIS) and approved of transferring elements from these systems to the medical sector [19, 33]. Analyses of the causes of accidents, derived from these reporting systems, brought to light that we should predominantly focus on error sources found on the organizational level. This root cause analysis model is then transferred to medical organizational structures.

5.4 Error classification

There exists a plethora of taxonomies to describe erroneous human behavior. In this context, we mention in passing the taxonomy after Rasmussen [34], which discriminates between three levels of human action:

1. skill-based action
2. rule-based action
3. knowledge-based action

Skill-based errors are those that occur when carrying out actions in which one is, in principle, fully competent. Rule-based errors are caused by inadequate information about the system's functional characteristics, leading to the application of incorrect rules of conduct. Knowledge-based errors develop due to lack of knowledge or due to inadequate application of acquired knowledge [35].

From this basis, Reason's "Generic Error Modeling System" (GEMS) tries to develop an integrated picture of error mechanisms on all three levels of action.

Unsafe actions and active failure usually have direct ramifications [36]. In contrast, the causes of latent failure can often be found on a higher organizational level and, in combination with other local, causative factors, may lead to system breakdown [19, 36]. Latent errors can often only be recognized after systematic analysis. Since latent errors imply holes in the system of safety barriers and thus pave the way for active errors, a prophylactic approach must be taken. Active errors are highly visible and hence have immediate consequences.

Since serious incidents and complications are rare, their analysis has only limited systemic impact on patient safety. Hence, it is more useful to analyze near-misses, critical incidents, rule violations, and malfunctions, which occur with much higher incidence.

As early as 1931, Heinrich [37] analyzed 550,000 accidents and discovered that for every deadly accident, 29 accidents with injuries and 300 potential accidents with a high risk of injuries were recorded. According to Heinrich's domino theory, accidents proceed along a natural chain of sequential events, each following a logical, quasi-deterministic chronological order. In his words: "The occurrence of a preventable injury is the natural culmination of a series of events or circumstances, which invariably occur in a fixed and logical order".

This ratio of near-misses to moderate injuries to major injuries is now known as the "300:29:1 ratio" and is cited in the literature in numerous variations on an iceberg model of stages of error escalation.

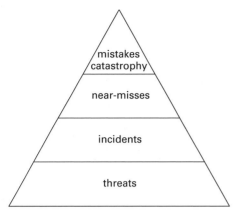

Fig. 5.1: Iceberg model [37]

The extended base of the iceberg consists of latent errors and incidents. Medical complications and actual catastrophes, such as amputating the wrong breast or operating on the wrong joint, only form the tip of the iceberg [37]. Critical incidents bear a potential for uncovering holes in a hospital's safety barriers. Damage occurs only once various unwanted events coincide and the chain of events penetrates through multiple safety holes, stacked on top of each other like holes in a Swiss cheese. This has often been visualized as the Swiss Cheese Model.

5.5 The JCAHO patient safety event taxonomy

As described earlier, by now, several projects have been started which target definition and classification of medical errors and near-misses [38, 39]. However, these models are often geared towards specific medical disciplines and specialisms, e.g., transfusion medicine [40], pharmacotherapy [41–43], and primary care [44, 45]. Most existing taxonomies were developed in relative isolation from classification schemes for other specific medical specialisms. Patient safety reporting systems differ in design and in their capability to define, count, and track adverse events [46]. There often exist disparate data fields, contradicting terminologies, and conflicting patient safety classification schemes, characteristics, and uses, which taken together make standardization difficult. There exists no standard for determining which events must be recorded and reported [47, 48].

The "Patient Safety Event Taxonomy", a method of classification developed by the JCAHO (Joint Commission of Accreditation of Healthcare Organizations), is based on evaluations of existing taxonomies and reporting systems and on feedback from its intended user base [49].

1. Impact—the outcome or effects of medical error and systems failure, commonly referred to as harm to the patient.
2. Type—the implied or visible processes that were faulty or failed.
3. Domain—the characteristics of the setting in which an incident occurred and the type of individuals involved.

4. Cause—the factors and agents that led to an incident.
5. Prevention and mitigation—the measures taken or proposed to reduce incidence and effects of adverse occurrences [49].

"Impact" comprises three subclassifications that discriminate between 18 different types of effects. "Type" includes three levels addressing communication, patient management, and clinical performance, each with its own subclassifications. "Domain" includes the types of health care professionals commonly involved in patient care and patient demographics in a variety of health care settings where adverse events may occur. The principal nodes of "Cause" consist of two subclassifications: systemic failures (process/structure) and human failures. In the final category, three different types of prevention and mitigation are identified: universal, selective, and indicated.

The analytical framework of the JCAHO patient safety event taxonomy provides an organized approach to the retrospective process of identifying the factors (causes) that contribute to system failures (type) and adverse events or to identify potential risk factors, on the basis of which preventive strategies (prevention) and corrective actions (mitigation) may be devised, which help protect the patient (in a domain) from harm (impact).

5.6 Reporting systems as tools to aid safety culture and risk management

Effective medical error and risk management depends on reporting errors and near-misses. The purpose of (mandatory) error reporting systems is to collect reports of severe incidents that have led to visible damage. A Critical Incidents Reporting System (CIRS), on the other hand, anonymously aggregates voluntary, confidential reports of near-misses, lower error escalation stages, and minor cases of complications or patient damage. In a CIRS, in contrast to classic error analysis, the actual damage, if any, plays only a secondary role, based on the idea that error analysis after the fact is too late to be of benefit in cases where actual damage occurred. Structured reporting, review, and continuous analysis of near-misses are essential for preventing severe damage, because all-important prevention strategies derive from their study. Modern hospitals are service providers or "enterprises of special kind". In addition, a lot of properties of the services provided by a hospital are related to issues involving experience and trust and display a more or less pronounced asymmetry of information distribution, away from the patient. Due to the complexity, indeterminism, and nonlinearity of the way diseases progress, the various services are highly heterogeneous, implying limited potential for standardization, which in turn requires a large amount of flexibility from all participants [50]. Hence, hospitals provide complex, personalized services, dominated by individual humans and facilitated by a high degree of integration of human and technical potential. These dimensions of complexity are characterized by a large number of service components. Other characteristics are their heterogeneity and the involvement of more than one individual on the one hand and a high degree of personalization on the other hand. Hence, it may be quite problematic to assess quality of service solely by medical outcome. As before, the spectrum of criteria to measure quality of medical outcome against the backdrop of evidence-based medicine is relatively small. Transparency is the best universal indicator for good quality of medical service.

CIRS and its connected open safety culture guarantee a high degree of transparency and quality improvement within the framework of comprehensive risk management. Hence, as mentioned earlier, systematic collection of near-misses was initiated already at an early stage, in particular in the English-speaking world. This may be contrasted with Germany, where, not that long ago, medical errors were largely considered as an aspect of personal responsibility [51] and error prevention used to mean demanding increasing perfectionism from the staff. Employees who reported mistakes had to be prepared to face punitive action. As a logical consequence any errors that occurred were swept under the rug. Errors, however, are caused by multiple factors. They often have systemic causes and come at the end of a chain of near-misses and latent errors. Hence, anonymous, voluntary collection of critical incidents will help eliminate error sources and weak spots in the system before serious complications can develop. By disposing of the fear of punitive action, the previous "culture of blame" may be replaced by a "culture of safety" [52]. Incident report systems must be easy to apply and comprehensibly structured. The use of standardized reply forms has stood the test. Accurate data acquisition requires that critical incidents and adverse events are documented as early as possible. In 80% of cases that were reported within three days, an accurate description of the event and its concomitant circumstances was possible. It is also essential for success to ensure regular feedback on the review of critical incidents and adverse events, and the ensuing changes to workflow, working standards, guidelines, and procedural instructions, on the basis of the error sources that could be identified. Leape [53] summarized the essential characteristics of an effective reporting system as follows:

Tab. 5.1: Characteristics of effective reporting systems [53–57]

1. Facilitates continuous optimization of an affirmative safety culture within an organization

2. Absence of punitive action towards the respondent and other people involved (anonymous reporting, legal protection of privacy)

3. System functioning independent of established hierarchy, i.e., reports are not sent to managing staff (heads of departments or staff positions)

4. System-relevant
   • Accessible to all relevant persons (e.g., physicians and nurses)
   • Uncomplicated reporting (for everyone, everywhere)
   • Educating the respondents about human factors

5. Room for free text, since this is where the focal point of the information can be found

6. Prompt feedback to the respondent (input, analysis, consequences)

7. Review by (interdisciplinary) experts on error analysis involving human factors, followed by warnings, instructions, and measures taken on their basis. If necessary, on site downstream analysis, e.g., root cause analysis (RCA) or failure mode effects analysis (FMEA)

8. Prompt implementation of suggested improvements. (If the reporting system does not allow for quick reaction, or does not have sufficient resources at its disposal, frustration will paralyze employees' readiness to file reports)

9. Monitoring the effectiveness of the improvements made

10. Organizational encouragement of reporting (working time, absence of internal punitive action, other rewards and incentives).

The WHO Draft Guidelines for Adverse Event Reporting and Learning Systems summarizes some practical methods for generating knowledge, along with theoretical underpinning and practical tips for designing reporting systems [58].
Four core principles underlie these guidelines:

- The fundamental role of reporting systems is to enhance patient safety through learning from failures that occur within the healthcare system.
- Reporting must be free from punitive action towards respondents. They should not be punished or suffer other ill effects due to their reporting.
- Reporting is only of value if it leads to a constructive response. At minimum, this entails feedback of the findings from data analysis. Ideally, it also includes recommendations for changes to processes and healthcare systems.
- Meaningful analysis, learning, and dissemination of any lessons learned require professional expertise, in conjunction with other human and financial resources. The agency that receives the reports must be competent in disseminating information, recommending changes, and guiding the development of solutions.

The primary purpose of patient safety reporting systems is to learn from experience. It is important to note that reporting does not by itself improve safety. It is the response to reports which effects changes. Within a healthcare institution, reporting a serious event or a serious "near-miss" must trigger an in-depth investigation to identify the underlying systemic failure, and it must initiate efforts to redesign the systems so that recurrence can be prevented.

In the United States, the USP's MEDMARX℠ system receives thousands of confidential reports on medication errors and adverse drug events from participating healthcare organizations. This (classified) data is then provided as feedback to healthcare organizations, together with benchmarks compiled from the entire database as well as their own prior experience in order to identify targets for improvement and to enable progress monitoring.

Accountability reporting systems assign responsibility to healthcare organizations by requiring reporting of serious incidents and by discouraging continuation of unsafe practices by handing out citations, penalties, and sanctions [59]. In these systems, reporting may also be educational if the lessons learned are widely shared [60]. However, the threat of sanctions may cause healthcare organizations to be reluctant in reporting events if they can be swept under the rug.

Since the absence of punitive measures is an almost indispensible condition, anonymous reporting systems are preferred. They may be open to a large group of respondents, such as the German nationwide PaSOS-System [61], but may also be limited to individual clinics and departments in order to obtain a clearer picture of location-specific features [11, 62, 63].

Ideally, internal reporting systems work in conjunction with external systems by identifying and analyzing events that warrant forwarding to external agencies.

Reports may be filed by both physicians and nurses, but patient reports may also be an important source of information which can help improve a hospital's safety culture. For example, a patient may develop complications from surgery after discharge from hospital. They may report, e.g., that treatment in another hospital was necessary to remove a stone in the ductus hepatocholedocheus, left behind after a prior cholecystectomy. Reports may be submitted via email, internet, intranet, or anonymously over telephone. Web-based Systems are able to centralize and aggregate multiple reports in a highly structured database. Reports also may be highly structured and ask for specific information. Events based on commonly accepted data elements, such as the classification of medication errors as wrong medication, wrong dose, wrong frequency, etc., may be readily organized into a standardized reporting format. The use of free text fields facilitates providing multiple answers or comments. The recorded information must include the type of incident, the time it occurred, its suspected cause, and, optionally, an estimate of the hazards to which the patient was exposed. In a hospital or a network of clinics, the reporting system may, for example, collect separate reports from each medical specialism, e.g., orthopedics, visceral surgery, thoracic surgery, plastic surgery, etc., which may then be forwarded to the commission responsible for the department's error management or to an interdisciplinary working group. Reports may then be analyzed and classified according to type of error, cause of error, and type of risk. Most of all, prompt review is mandated so that recurring critical incidents and adverse events can be identified and solutions may be implemented.

The main target of any reporting system is an early recognition of system-level weaknesses and malfunctions, so as to induce improvement on various systemic, organizational levels. Anonymous reporting systems mainly target incidents and near-misses that have relevance to patient safety. A somewhat different method is direct incident analysis, called "Failure Modes and Effects Analysis", which identifies and analyzes each single step of the process for potential sources of error and formulates and implements changes to the system. Another important tool is to employ independent experts to monitor processes in the hospital. Objectivity may be increased by integrating video analysis into the monitoring process. A so-called "safety walkaround" is a process in which a group of senior leaders visits individual units within a healthcare organization and interviews frontline staff about specific events and possible solutions. Subsequently, the hospital's patient safety team, in cooperation with the medical staff, can develop solution strategies.

Besides publications on medical malpractice in scientific journals, discharge codes, assigned after discharge from inpatient care provide an important source of information.

In the United States, the Agency for Healthcare Research and Quality (AHRQ) has developed a list of specific discharge codes, called Patient Safety Indicators (PSI), that are strongly correlated with "problems that patients experience as a result of exposure to the healthcare system and that are likely amenable to prevention" [57, 64]. The United States Veterans Health Administration National Surgical Quality Improvement Program (NSQIP) exemplifies variants of surveillance on a much larger scale [65].

After implementation of the NSQIP, the mortality rate after surgery decreased by 27% and complications by 45%, over the ten year period 1999–2000 [66]. Program leaders attribute most of these reductions to changes that hospitals implemented in response to feedback from the data.

The NSQIP's success in reducing adverse events and mortality rates can be attributed to five factors:

1. For all patients, not just those with complications, data collection is integrated into daily routine.
2. Designated, trained individuals are responsible for the data collection.
3. The results are risk-adjusted.

4. Hospitals receive feedback in the form of site-specific data and comparison with their peers.
5. Outcomes are monitored by a central authority, authorized to conduct visitations and require changes.

The WHO Draft Guidelines for adverse Event Reporting and Learning Systems contain a comprehensive review of reporting systems in use throughout the world. Most countries have voluntary, anonymous reporting systems. Existing national reporting systems display large variability in financial support, participation, and function. In the following we mention a few examples.

Examples: In February 2004, the National Reporting and Learning System (NRLS) was launched in England and Wales by the National Patient Safety Agency (NPSA) to promote an open reporting culture.

Patient safety incidents subject to reporting are defined as "any unintended or unexpected incident that could have or did lead to harm to one or more patients receiving NHS-funded healthcare". Reports are anonymous, although an NHS Trust identifier is maintained. Any staff or patient names are removed before data is entered into the database.

Healthcare organizations that use electronic risk management systems can submit reports to the NRLS by directly linking them from the local system. The NPSA has worked with local risk management software vendors to insure compatibility and consistency of user interfaces. Weekly, around 10,000 reports are submitted to the NRLS. The NSPA works together with every affected party, to help integrate their own dataset into that of the NRLS [67].

Adverse events are categorized according to type and may be subdivided into groups with descriptors such as, e.g., wrong quantity, wrong route, etc. in the case of medication events. Reports are aggregated and analyzed, and auxiliary input from clinical experts is obtained to help understand the frequency with which each type of patient safety incident occurs and to search for patterns, trends, and underlying contributory factors.

In the Netherlands, most hospitals and other healthcare organizations have nonpunitive, voluntary reporting systems in place. There also exists a mandatory system for reporting serious adverse events that result in permanent injury or death. There exists no standardized classification scheme for shared use by individual hospital systems, meaning that there is no nationwide data aggregation.

The Swedish healthcare law of 1997 requires each medical institution to have a quality control system in place, which most medical institutions have implemented in different forms. Systems are regulated by decrees issued by the National Board of Health and Welfare (NBHW).

Reporting and learning systems are part of regulations requiring hospitals to investigate serious events and to redesign their systems. All reports submitted to the NBHW are publicly accessible, but all patients' personal data is kept confidential.

The United States does not have a federal reporting system. However, 21 of the 50 states have mandatory reporting systems in place, many of which have been there for decades. All of these require mandatory reporting of unexpected deaths, and several also require reporting wrong-site surgery. Beyond this, definitions of what constitutes a reportable event vary widely. Reports of serious events may prompt an on-site investigation by a state's health department.

The Institute for Safe Medication Practices (ISMP) is a national, confidential reporting system for medication errors that distributes hazard alerts and other medication safety information to 600,000 providers every other week. The ISMP focuses on reports of adverse drug events and risks related to the delivery and management of medication. Information is classified according to 10 key elements. In the identification of hazards, human expertise is exploited by engaging a group of experts to observe recurrent reports and work together closely to apply their knowledge to assessing the urgency of a problem. A rapid turnaround permits numerous alerts so that an overall analysis for prioritization is not required.

In 1996, the Joint Commission implemented a Sentinel Event Reporting System, designed to enable healthcare organizations to identify and learn from sentinel events and their prevention strategies. The system is voluntary and confidential. The accreditation status of any reporting organization remains unaffected, as long as it takes resolute action to prevent future recurrence.

Sentinel events subject to reporting are defined as events that result in an unanticipated death or major permanent loss of function, unrelated to the natural course of the patient's illness or underlying condition. The following are also considered sentinel events even if patient death or major loss of function in the sense mentioned above did not occur: suicide of any individual receiving care, treatment, or services in settings with nonstop availability of medical personnel or within 72 hours after discharge, unanticipated infant death, abduction of any individual receiving care, treatment or services releasing an infant to the wrong family, rape, hemolytic transfusion reactions involving administration of blood products with major blood group incompatibilities, surgery on the wrong individual or body part, and unintentionally retained foreign bodies after surgery or other procedures.

At regular intervals, based on their database and their collaborations with experts, the JCAHO selects a particular event type and issues a Sentinel Event Alert describing the event itself, its causes, and preventive strategies that were gathered from various organizations.

The United States Pharmacopoeia's MedMARxSM is a voluntary system designed to identify hazards and system vulnerabilities, identify best practices, and gather information that helps support the USP's role in devising standards. Reports include adverse drug events, near-misses, and other errors, that may all be submitted to MedMARXSM.

MedMARXSM accepts reports submitted by healthcare professionals, organizations, and patients. Since its introduction in 1998, more than 900 healthcare facilities have contributed over 630,000 medication error reports [Personal communication with J. Silverstone National Patient Safety Foundation email list serve, editor. 4-20-2004]. Currently, it receives approximately 20,000 reports each month [Personal communication with D. Cousins 5-19-2004], corresponding to about 20 per month for each of their 900 healthcare facilities.

The Australian Incident Monitoring System (AIMS) was founded in 1993 as an extension of the Anaesthesia AIMS, established in 1987. The AIMS' objective is to promote education on newly emerged hazards, trends, risk factors, and any contributing factors.

AIMS is designed to process a wide range of events, including predefined "sentinel" events, any adverse event, near-misses, equipment failures, newly emerged hazards, and specific events such as suicide and abduction. The AIMS accepts and classifies information originating from any source, including incident reports, sentinel events, root cause analysis, coroner's reports, consumer reports, and reviews of morbidity and mortality rates.

The classification system used by the AIMS is perhaps the most highly developed of any known reporting system and comprises more than a million permutations of terms for describing incidents or adverse events. The purpose of this classification scheme is to translate information about individual incidents into a common language and to create an electronic record which may be compared with other records and can be analyzed as part of a larger dataset. The latest classification is based on Professor Runciman's Generic Reference Model (GRM). The GRM is based on Reason's model for failure in complex systems [68].

The GRM consists of contributing factors (environmental, organizational, and human factors, characteristics of the incident, agents involved in the incident), incident details (type, component, person(s) involved, time of the incident, time of detection, method of detection, preventability), factors that minimize or aggravate outcome or consequences, and consequences for patient and healthcare organization.

In Japan, the Ministry of Health, Labor and Welfare requires hospitals to have internal reporting systems in place. The Japan Council for Quality Health Care collects voluntary incident reports. In 2004, it implemented a national reporting system, in which reporting is mandatory for teaching hospitals and voluntary for others.

Reporting systems exist on three levels: systems limited to the individual hospital or health facility, voluntary systems in various forms, such as accreditation bodies for hospitals and research groups, and a national level with mandatory reporting.

Subject to reporting are patient injuries, sometimes referred to as adverse events, along with near-misses and equipment malfunctions. Any hospital or healthcare organization may voluntarily report to the accrediting bodies. Reporting to the Japan Council for Quality Health Care is mandatory. All information is reported in electronic form.

Cases that are deemed of particular importance are evaluated individually. Otherwise, reports are aggregated for statistical analysis (no further details are available). The Japan Council for Quality Health Care produces summaries of event reports, which are then released to healthcare providers and to the public.

As of February 1, 2011, it has been possible for all employees of the surgical department in the Swiss city of Chur to anonymously or openly report any incident, independent of its severity, to a central agency with use of standardized reply forms. Data is continuously accumulated and presented once a month in an internal quality meeting [69].

The German Alliance for Patient Safety, founded as late as 2005, strives to set up a framework for action towards patient safety. In analogy to examples in other countries, in particular in the UK and Switzerland, Germany is installing a rapidly increasing number of incident reporting systems. Besides various in-house systems, there exist several systems that have a scope reaching beyond local institutes as well as discipline-specific and internet-based systems.

A working group from the German Alliance for Patient Safety has developed a comprehensive introductory manual for the use of CIRSs:

- Aktionsbündnis Patientensicherheit (2006): Empfehlung zur Einführung von CIRS im Krankenhaus. http://www.aktionsbuendnis-patientensicherheit.de/apsside/07-07-25-CIRS-Handlungsempfehlung.pdf (07.12.07).

Several German medical societies offer their members access to CIRSs specific to their discipline. These include the German Society for surgery (DGCH), the German Society for Anesthesiology and Intensive Care (DGAI), the German Society for Gynecology and Obstetrics (DGGG), and the German Association of Pain Studies (DGSS).

The various systems feature different sets of questions. Each has predefined answer categories. Additional free text fields are available to note further details.

CIRS medical Germany was instituted by the German Medical Association and the German National Association of Statutory Health Insurance Physicians, as part of their measures for quality insurance.

The German CIRS Network for Hospitals is a reporting system for hospital-related incidents with relevance to patient safety.

Tab. 5.2: Incident reporting systems

www.cirsmedical.de	Critical incident reporting system of the German Medical Association, organized by the German Agency for Quality in Medicine and provided by the GMA and the National Association of Statutory Health Insurance Physicians
www.pasis.de	Patient safety system of the University of Tübingen, organized by the city's Center for Patient Safety and Simulations, the Clinic for Anesthesiology and Intensive Care, and the University Clinic.
www.jeder-fehler-zaehlt.de	Error reporting and educational system for general practices, organized by the Frankfurt University Institute for General Medicine and supported by the Federal Ministry of Health
www.pasos-ains.de	Patient Safety Organizational System of the German Society of Anesthesiologists and Intensive Care Medicine and the Federal Association of Anesthesiologists.
www.dgss.org	Critical incident reporting system of the German Association of Pain Studies, DGSS.
www.cirs-notfallmedizin. de/home.html	Critical incident reporting and risk management system in preclinical emergency medicine, organized by the Department of Anesthesiology, Intensive Care and Emergency Medicine of the University of Kempten.
www.dgch.de/cirs/index.html	Critical incident reporting system of the German Society for Surgery
www.kritische-ereignisse.de.de	Learning from critical incidents: error reporting and educational system for geriatric care of the German Society for the Aged-Wilhelmine-Lübke Foundation, Cologne.

5.6.1. CIRS as an aspect of risk management

A CIRS deals with risks and generates risk-related knowledge that cannot be provided by other information systems. Recognizing risk constellations is, however, only the first step in the error prevention process within the framework of in-house risk management. CIRSs are just one particular tool employed in risk management and may not be equated with the whole domain. They are not by themselves sufficient for structured processing and sustainable, methodical mitigation of near-misses. In realizing this, e.g., the Hannover medical academy has extended the classic CIRS by introducing two additional components (the "3 Be-System®"). Despite the increasing number of patients treated, a significant decline of the number of incidents involving patient damage could be achieved with the help of structured processing of submitted reports and methodical mitigation of reported risks [70]. CIRSs as well as risk management must become part of the DNA of every person involved. A CIRS is not a bureaucracy but demands active participation. Availability of external or internal reporting systems will initially not yet influence patient safety directly. Stepwise fortification of safety culture can only be achieved with system-oriented analyses, by providing feedback to respondents and by devising usable improvement strategies. One limitation of CIRS is that it does not allow for quantitative evaluation of the incidence of adverse events. They also often show the paradoxical effect that, once a reporting system is in place, the number of reported incidents increases. An increase in the monthly number of reported errors may reflect the functioning of patient safety systems in the hospital, but may also mean that employees are more highly motivated to report errors because they are now convinced that their reports are adequately dealt with and that they lead to actual quality improvements. Reporting every single incident is, however, not useful because this would rapidly generate an almost unmanageably large data volume.

For example, in Pennsylvania hospitals are only required to report all serious events, incidents, and hospital-acquired infections.

In 2004, the UK's National Patient Safety Agency (NPSA) established a national incident reporting system. In 2006, already more than one million reports had been filed. In Pennsylvania, ca. 400,000 reports were filed. Ways are being sought to cope with such massive volumes of data. Pennsylvania, for example, publishes a quarterly newsletter that discusses essential adverse events obtained from the reporting system [71].

One particular method, that is, used to identify certain types of errors, in particular medication errors, utilizes so-called "trigger tools". Many medication errors leave behind traces, e.g., antidotes used after overdosing anticoagulant drugs. Another highly valuable tool is to organize so-called "Morbidity/Mortality meetings" (M+M meetings), where critical incidents and actual errors are presented to a large selection of coworkers. Regrettably, such meetings are only held regularly in about half of all German hospitals. However, in the surgical disciplines, M+M meetings often focus only on the human aspects of errors that occurred and system-related aspects are addressed insufficiently. The chairman must possess a large amount of empathy and intuition, in order to prevent these meetings from devolving into mere "shame-and-blame" sessions. In the USA, the content of M+M meetings is protected by law, as long as it is an integrated part of quality control [72].

The process of establishing nationwide structures for effective risk management is still under development and as of yet far away from completion. In establishing safety culture within a hospital, one should be guided by Leape's observation that: "The problem is not bad people in health care - it is that good people are working in bad systems that need to be made safer" [73].

5.7 Summary

The medical sector must develop a nationwide systemic safety culture similar to other high-security branches such as the industrial sector and the aviation industry. To achieve this, its traditional dogmas must first be surmounted. It is especially important to change one's mental concept of errors and stop regarding them as individual failure subject to punishment. The current culture of blame must be supplanted by a change of perspective based on the realization that errors can happen whenever and wherever people work together. Errors must be regarded as sources of knowledge, and it is of prime importance to learn lessons from them. Based on this realization, numerous systemic approaches towards developing safety culture have been designed.

References

[1] Jahoda, G. Do we need a Concept of Culture? In: Journal of Cross-Cultural Psychology, 1984, Vol. 15, No 2, p 139–151.
[2] Health and Safety Commission: Third Report: Organizing for Safety, ACSNI, Study Group on Human Factors - HMSO 1993; London.
[3] Reason, JT. Human error. Cambridge University Press, 1990; New York.
[4] Reason, JT. Human error: models and management. BMJ 2000; 320:768–770.
[5] Kirstein, H. Der Einfluss Deming auf die Entrichtung des Total Quality Management (TQM), 1994, München.
[6] Salzgeber, F. Kunden- und Prozessorientierung in Versicherungsunternehmen, Karlsruhe 1996; 209–228.
[7] Crosby, PB. Qualitätsmanagement, 2000, Wien.
[8] Eckes, G. The Six Sigma Revolution: How General Electric and Others Turned Process into Profits, 2001; New York.
[9] Harry, M, Schroeder, R, Hohmann, BJ. Six Sigma: Prozesse optimieren, Null-Fehler-Qualität schaffen, Rendite radikal steigern, 2005; 3rd ed. Frankfurt a.M.
[10] Pande, PS, Neumann, RP, Cavanagh, RR. The Six Sigma way: How GE, Motorola and other top companies are horning their performance. McGraw-Hill Professional, 2000; New York.
[11] Hübler, M, Möllemann, A, Metzler, H. et al. Fehler und Fehlermeldesysteme in der Anästhesie. Anaesthetist 2007; 56:1067–1072.
[12] Park, K. Human error. In: Salvendy G (ed). Handbook of human factor and ergonomics. Willey, New York, 1997; pp 150–173.
[13] Keenan, V, Kerr, W, Sherman, W. Psychological Climate and Accidents in an Automotive Plant, In: Journal of Applied Psychology 1951; Vol 35, No 2, p 108–111.
[14] Coquelle, IJ, Cura, B, Fourest, B. Safety, Culture and Quality System. In: Carino, A, Weiman, G. (ed). Proceedings of the International Topical Meeting on Safety Culture in Nuclear Installations; American Nuclear Society of Austria, Vienna, 1995; p 193–202.
[15] Cox, S, Cox, T. The structure of Employee Attitudes to Safety: An European Example. In: Work and Stress, 1991; Vol 5, No 2, p 189–201.
[16] Cox, S, Flin, RF. Safety culture: Philosopher's Stone or Man of Straw? In: Work and Stress, 1998; Vol 12, No 3, p 189–201.
[17] Pidgeon, N. Safety Culture: Key Theoretical Issues. In: Work and Stress, 1998; Vol 12, No 3, p 202–216.
[18] Zhang, H, Wiegmann, DG, Thaden, TL. et al. Safety Culture: A Concept in Chaos? In: Human Factors and Ergonomics Society (ed). Proceedings of the 46th Annual Human Factors and Ergonomics Society Meeting, Santa Monica 2002; p 1404–1408.

[19] Löber, N. Fehler und Fehlerkultur im Krankenhaus. Gabler Verlag Wiesbaden 2012.

[20] Flaatten, H. The importance of ICN Culture. In: Chiche, J.-D., Moreno, R., Putensen, C. et al. (ed). Patient safety and Quality of Care in Intensive Care Medicine, Berlin, 2009; p. 87–91.

[21] Barach, P, Small, SD. Reporting and preventing medical mishaps: lessons from non-medical near miss reporting systems. BMJ 2000; 320:759–763.

[22] Klinect, JR, Wilhelm, JA, Helmreich, R. Threat and error management: data from line operations safety audits. Proceedings of the 10th International symposium on aviation psychology. Ohio State University, Columbus 1999; pp 683–688.

[23] Kohn, LT, Corrigan, JM, Donaldson, MS. (ed): Committee on Quality in Health Care; Institute of Medicine: to err is human. Building a safer health system. National Academy Press 1999; Washington.

[24] McWilson, LR, Runciman, WB, Gibberd, RW. et al. The quality in Australian health care study. Med J Aust 1995; 163:458–471.

[25] Vincent, C, Neale, G, Woloshynowych, M. Adverse events in British hospitals: preliminary retrospective record review, BMJ 2001; 322:517–519.

[26] Zegers, M, de Bruijne, MC, Wagner, C. et al. Adverse events and potentially preventable deaths in Dutch hospitals: results of a retrospective patient record review study. Qual Saf Health Care 2009; 18:297–302.

[27] Soop, M, Fryksmark, U, Köster, M, Haglund, B. The incidence of adverse events in Swedish hospitals: a retrospective medical record review study. Int J Qual Health Care 2009; 21: 285–291.

[28] Baker, GR, Norton, PG, Flintoft, V. et al. The Canadian adverse events study: the incidence of adverse events study: the incidence of adverse events among hospital patients in Canada. CMAJ 2004; 170:1678–1186.

[29] Schimmel, EM. The hazards of hospitalisation. Ann Intern Med 1964; 60:100–110. In: Cohen, D. Maßnahmen zur Verbesserung der Patientensicherheit. Bundesgesundheitsbl 2011; 54:171–175.

[30] Rybowiak, V, Garst, H, Frese, M. et al. Error Orientation Questionnaire (EOQ): Reliability, Validity, and Different Language Equivalence, In: Journal of Organizational Behaviour 1999; Vol 20, no 4, p 527–547.

[31] Baer, M, van Dyck, C, Frese, M. et al. Organizational Errors Management Culture and its Impact on Performance: A two-study-Replication, In: Journal of Applied Psychology 2005; Vol 90, no 6, p 1228–1240.

[32] Schüttelkopf, E. Erfolgsstrategie Fehlerkultur. In: Ebner, G, Heimerl, P, Schüttelkopf, EM (ed). Fehler-Lernen-Unternehmen: Wie Sie die Fehlerkultur und Lernreife Ihrer Organisation wahrnehmen und gestalten. Frankfurt a.M. 2008; p. 151–314.

[33] Reason, JT. Managing the Risks of Organizational Accidents, Aldershot 1997.

[34] Rasmussen, J. Human Errors: A Taxonomy for Describing Human Malfunction in Industrial Installations. In: Journal of Occupational Accidents, 1982; Vol 4, no 2-4, p. 311–333.

[35] Reason, JT. Menschliches Versagen: Psychologische Risikofaktoren und moderne Technologien, Heidelberg 1994.

[36] Reason, JT. Understanding Adverse Events: Human factors. In: Quality and Safety in Health Care, 1995; Vol 4, no 2, p. 80–89.

[37] Heinrich, HW, Granniss, ER. Industrial Accident Prevention, 4th ed. 1959, New York. Cited in: Löber, N. Fehler und Fehlerkultur im Krankenhaus. Gabler Verlag Wiesbaden 2012.

[38] Runciman, WB, Helps, SC, Sexton, EJ. et al. A classification for incidents and accidents in the healthcare system. J Qual Clin Pract 1998; 18:199–211.

[39] Elder, NC, Dovey, SM. Classification of medical errors and preventable adverse events in primary care: A synthesis of the literature. J Fam Pract 2002; 51:927–932.

[40] Kaplan, HS, Battles, JB, van der Schaaf, TW, Shea, CE, Mercer, SQ. Identification and classification of the causes of events in transfusion medicine. Transfusion 1998; 38:1071–1081.

[41] Dunn, EB, Wolfe, JJ. Medication error classification and avoidance. Hosp Pharm 1997; 32:860–865.

[42] National Coordinating Council for Medication Error Reporting and Prevention, USA. NCC MERP Taxonomy of Medication Errors. 1998. http://www.nccmerp.org/taxo0731. pdf Accessed 3 June 2003.

[43] Betz, RP, Levy, HB. An interdisciplinary method of classifying and monitoring medication errors. Am J Hosp Pharm 1985; 42:1724–1732.

[44] Makeham, MA, Dovey, SM, County, M, Kidd, MR. An international taxonomy for errors in general practice: a pilot study. Med J Aus 2002; 177:62–63.

[45] Dovey, SM, Meyers, DS, Phillips, RL. et al. A preliminary taxonomy of medical errors in family practice. Qual Saf Health Care 2002; 11:233–38.

[46] Implementation Planning Study for the Integration of Medical Event Reporting Input and Data Structure for Reporting to AHRQ, CDC, CMS, and FDA. Medstat Report submitted to AHRQ, 2002.

[47] Weingart, SN, Wilson, RM, Gibberd, RW, Harrison, B. Epidemiology of medical error. BMJ 2000; 320:730.

[48] University of California at San Francisco-Stanford University. Evidence-based Practice Center. Making Health Care Safer: A Critical Analysis of Patient Safety Practices. Report No. AHRQ 01-E508. Rockville, MD: Agency for Healthcare Research and Quality, 2001.

[49] Chang, A, Schyve, PM, Croteau, RJ. et al. The JCAHO patient safety event taxonomy: a standardized terminology and classification schema for near misses and adverse events. International Journal for Quality in Health Care 2005; Vol 17, No 2: p 95–105.

[50] Düllinger, F. Krankenhaus-Management im Spannungsfeld zwischen Patientenorientierung und Rationalisierung: Probleme und Gestaltungsmöglichkeiten des Business Reengineering in der Krankenhaus-Praxis, München 1996.

[51] Köbberling, J. Das Critical Incident Reporting System (CIRS) als Mittel zur Qualitätsverbesserung in der Medizin. Med Klin 2005; 100:143–148.

[52] Rall, M. Patient safety and errors in medicine: development, prevention and analyses of incidents. Anaesthesiol Intensivmed Notfallmed Schmerzther 2001; 36(6):321–330.

[53] Leape, LL. Reporting of adverse events. N Engl J Med 2002; 347(20):1633–1638.

[54] Rall, M, Gaba, DM. Human performance and patient safety. In: Miller, RD (ed). Miller's anesthesia. Elsevier Churchill Livingston, Philadelphia, 2005; p. 3021–3071.

[55] Rall, M, Martin, J, Geldner, G. et al. Charakteristika effektiver Incident-Reporting-Systeme zur Erhöhung der Patientensicherheit. Anaesthesiol Intensivmed 2006; 47:9–19.

[56] Stricker, E, Rall, M, Siegert, N. et al. Das Patienten-Sicherheits-Informations-System PaSIS. Ein internet-basiertes interaktives Meldesystem für negative und positive Ereignisse in der Anästhesie. Intensiv- und Notfallmedizin. In: Jäckel, A (ed). Telemedizinführer. Medizin-Forum 2006; Ober-Mörlen, p. 67–77.

[57] World Health Organization: WHO draft guidelines for adverse event reporting and learning systems. 2005; WHO/EIP/SPO/QPS/05.3, Geneva.

[58] World alliance for patient safety. WHO draft guidelines for adverse event reporting and learning systems – from information to action. http://www.who.int/patientsafety/events/05/ Reporting-Guidelines.pdf.

[59] Flowers, L, Riley, T. State-based mandatory reporting of medical errors. An analysis of the legal and policy issues. Portland, ME, National Academy for State Health Policy, 2001.

[60] Kohn, L, Corrigan, JM, Donaldson, MS. To err is human: Building a safer health system. Washington, DC, National Academy Press, 1999.

[61] Rall, M, Dieckmann, P., Stricker, E. Arbeitsgruppe Incident Reporting innerhalb des Forums Qualitätssicherung und Ökonomie des BDA und der DGAI. Patientensicherheits-Optimierungs-System (PaSOS) – Das neue bundesweite Incident-Reporting-System von DGAI/BDA. Anaesth Intensivmed 2006; 47:520–524.

[62] Hübler, M, Möllemann, A, Eberlein-Gonska, M. et al. Anonymes Meldesystem kritischer Ereignisse in der Anästhesie – Ergebnisse nach 18 Monaten. Anaesthesist 2006; 55:133–141.

[63] Möllemann, A, Eberlein-Gonska, M, Koch, T, Hübler, M. Klinisches Risikomanagement – Implementierung eines anonymen Fehlermeldesystems in der Anästhesie eines Universitätsklinikums. Anaesthesist 2005; 54:377–384.

[64] Mc Donald K. Measures of patient safety based on hospital administrative data: the patient safety indicators. Rockville, MD. Agency for Healthcare Research and Quality, 2002.

[65] Khuri, SF, Daley, J, Henderson, WG. The comparative assessment and improvement of quality of surgical care in the Department of Veterans Affairs. Archives of Surgery, 1998; 228: 491–507.

[66] Khuri, SF, Daley, J, Henderson, WG. The comparative assessment and improvement of quality of surgical care in the Department of Veterans Affairs. Archives of Surgery, 2002; 137:20–27.

[67] National Patient Safety Agency National Reporting and Learning System. Dataset (http://npsa.nhs.uk/dataset/dataset.asp.accessed) on 9 November 2005.

[68] Runciman, WB. Lessons from the Australian Patient Safety Foundation: setting up a national patient safety surveillance system – is this the right model? Quality and Safety in Health Care, 2002; 11:246–251.

[69] Missbach-Kroll, A, Nussbaumer, P, Kuenz, M. et al. Critical incident reporting system. Chirurg 2005; 76:868–875.

[70] Panzica, M, Krettek, C, Cartes, M. "Clinical Incident Reporting System" als Instrument des Risikomanagements für mehr Patientensicherheit. Unfallchirurg 2011; 114:758–767.

[71] Wachter, RM. Focus Patientensicherheit. ABW Wissenschaftsverlag 2008.

[72] Stewart, RM, Corneille, MG, Johnston, J. et al. Transparent and open discussion of errors does not increase malpractice risk in trauma patients. Ann Surg 2006; 243:645–651.

[73] Leape, LL. Error in Medicine. JAMA 1994; 272:1851–1857.

6 Ethical aspects of an open safety culture: towards a new physician-patient relationship in 21st century medicine

Since antiquity, the mission statement for physicians has been to provide care for patients. A physician is responsible for the "commodity" named "health". Health and wellbeing have always taken a prominent place in any culture's hierarchy of values and goods. Preserving a patient's health, providing care, and healing illnesses are occupations which, then and now, involve highest ethical standards, and were, not without reason, considered an "Art" by the ancient Greeks. For example Hippocrates described the "Medical Art" as follows: "As to diseases, make a habit of two things: to help, or at least to do no harm. The art has three factors, the disease, the patient, the physician. The physician is the servant of the art. The patient must co-operate with the physician in combating the disease." (Epidemics I, 11) [1]. In antiquity, as well as in the middle ages, disease was interpreted from a religious-spiritual perspective. Analogous to Asklepios, the Greek God of Medicine, Jesus of Nazareth was worshipped also as a physician ("Christus medicus").

Despite the widespread secularization of our western societies, the triumph of modern medicine, being firmly rooted in the natural sciences and modern technology, has caused medicine and, in particular, the contemporary physician as its representative to be ascribed quasi-titanic, i.e., superhuman abilities: all diseases will be cured once and for all, and humanity will never again have to live in fear of ill health. Despite the mechanization of the medical biosphere in our western cultural environment, despite the high degree of medicalization of an increasingly large number of cultures and of the way we reflect upon our own species, and despite the increasing dominance of economical and commercial factors, the modern physician, with his salutogenic approach, is still ascribed quasi-salutary capabilities, instilled in him by the exceptional power of modern science and biotechnological equipment. Against their will, modern physicians are confronted with an exaggerated image of their profession in the eyes of their patients. This leads patients to believe that an absolute zero-tolerance policy is seemingly the only acceptable standard. Nowadays, it is no longer sufficient that diseases be cured but, more importantly, people now expect lifelong health optimization. In addition, because that what nature and genetics provided us with is deemed insufficient, molecular-biological and biotechnological enhancements are expected to improve on the native equipment of the harangued, defective creature going under the name of Homo sapiens. This implies a view of health as a fundamental natural right, to be demanded from medicine, i.e., to be guaranteed by the physician with use of state of the art technology. This exaggerated view of the physician's role threatens to cause lasting damage to patient-physician relationships in modern medicine. The medical ethos is rooted in the act of prevention, i.e., it is an ethos that focuses on care, rather than cure, as in the Hippocratic Oath. In contrast, the modern basic ethical principle, which makes the patient's autonomy its focal point, was not known at the time and as such is not reflected in the Hippocratic Oath. The idea of autonomy as a basic principle of people's right to self-determination has its roots in the Enlightenment. According to Kant, only autonomy, as a reflection of free will, makes a human being an individual: "The autonomy of the will is the sole principle of all moral laws and of all duties which conform to them ... Thus the moral law expresses nothing else than the autonomy of the pure practical reason; that is, freedom; and this is itself the formal condition of all maxims, and on this condition only can they agree with the supreme practical law" [2]. Kant regarded autonomy as "[...] the basis of the dignity of human and of every rational nature." The lessons learned from the abuses of the medical Art in Germany, during the era of National Socialism, have been codified in the Nürnberg Codex from 1947, which makes any medical intervention subject to the patient's informed consent. Today, as it has been since antiquity, the principle of "non maleficence" has been one of medicine's fundamental principles. The following four principles, formulated in 1979 by Tom L. Beauchamp and James F. Childress, have had a profound influence on the medical-ethical discussion:

1. autonomy
2. to do no harm
3. to do good
4. justice [3]

In the 20th century, the will of any self-determined human being has increasingly gained the status of a supreme law. At the same time, the principle of prevention, as a relic from a more paternalistic age, has lost its value. This change has been accompanied by a paradigm shift from "beneficence model" to "autonomy model". In the United States, the idea of medicine as a unique occupational category has been associated with the concept of professionalism, as expressed by the tightly bound concepts of patient autonomy and accountability of the physician. E. Freidson declared medicine worthy to be labeled a "profession", because it self-regulates and is not subject to third party evaluation [4]. The hallmark of the physician's work as a practicing professional consists of ethically and medically appropriate patient care, based on the physician's best judgment. The way physicians have traditionally implemented this in their everyday work is characterized by the principle of autonomy. Accountability traditionally has been attributed to self, society, patient, profession, and to the medical ethical standards upheld in carrying out their profession [5].

Starting in the mid-20th century, the idyllic, paternalistic state of affairs, with its informal dependence of the patient on his physician, has drastically changed. Physicians used to feel comfortable in making decisions for their patients. Patient rights did not exist, and it was presumed that the physician acts in the patient's best interests. Therefore, liability issues had no place in this traditional, paternalistic image. Due to patients having increasingly better access to sources of information about general health and about their specific illness in particular, the doctor is no longer the sole, undisputed possessor of knowledge about diseases and their treatment. At the same time, a loosening and weakening of patient-physician relationships, previously tight and built on a foundation of trust and prevention, has developed and a political, social, and economical chasm has appeared, separating patient and physician. The patient no longer perceives the physician as a self-evident friend and mentor. Patients have started to search for information on best treatment options by themselves, and physicians have lost their role as uncontested guardians of knowledge and information. Since the mid-20th-century, patients have increasingly become consumers of "the product medicine" and their relationship with physicians ever more formal and distanced [6]. Increasingly isolated and alienated from its "customers", the medical profession complains of neurotic and overly demanding patients, who come to them prepared with lists of irritating questions – la maladie dú petit papier (the piece-of-paper disease) [7]. Such individuals were described in other sources as "hateful patients", "depending clingers", "entitled demanders", and "manipulative help rejecters" [8]. Individual responsibility for health preservation and prudent use of expensive medical treatment cannot be delegated. Healthcare systems are complex and require a considerable amount of personalized decision making. Consumers are increasingly forced to combat the spiraling cost of health insurance, choices between alternative treatments, nagging doubts about the quality of any care received, and conflicting evidence about the efficacy and safety of many procedures. When confronted with pain, discomfort, and feelings of fright and despair, patients seek information to help retain control over their body and to restore their life to normality. At this most vulnerable point in their lives, patients urgently need vital, life-sustaining information [9]. Katz argues that "the idea that doctors know what is in their patients' best interests and can therefore act on their behalf is so patently untrue that one can only marvel at the fervor with which the notion has been defended" [10].

The first of modern medicine's revolutions started in the 19th century, with general improvements in hygiene, cleaner and healthier water, and a better diet for broad levels of the population. The introduction of aseptic and antiseptic techniques, along with developments in anesthesiology, enabled previously life-threatening surgical procedures, such as amputations, laparotomies, or craniotomies, to be conducted almost painlessly, and with drastically reduced risk to the patient.

The second half of the 20th century has seen enormous scientific advances, in conjunction with advances in professional education and management, and immense resource investments to extend the provision of services. This second revolution has created powerful healthcare management systems, making the 20th century the century of physicians, clinics, and the medical industry. As illustrated by the contraceptive pill-scare in the United Kingdom and the striking misinformation of the European general public about pros and cons of cancer screening, it did not aim at creating knowledgeable patients [11]. Despite its great advances, the 20th century has left us with un-informed doctors and patients, unwarranted variations in how medicine is practiced, waste of resources, and problems with patient safety. Most countries can no longer afford such wasteful systems and the recent financial crises provide a unique opportunity for change: the time is ripe for a third revolution. Where the first revolution gave us clean water and the second introduced groundbreaking technical innovations to operating theatres, we are now standing on the threshold of a third medical revolution, which rings in a century of information, where the spotlight is on the fully informed and autonomous patient – the realization of the ancient democratic ideal. Citizens have the right to know the basic facts and carry a responsibility to base their healthcare decisions on the best evidence available [12]. This democratic ideal was, e.g., expressed by the second president of the United States, John Adams: "The preservation of the means of knowledge among the lowest ranks is of more importance to the public than all property of all the rich men in the country" [13].

Many doctors, and most patients, do not understand the available medical evidence. Seven "sins" contributing to this lack of knowledge have been identified: biased funding, biased reporting in medical journals, biased patient information pamphlets and media reports, conflicts of interest, defensive medicine, and medical curricula that fail to teach doctors how to interpret and understand healthcare statistics. Almost ten million US women have been screened for cervical cancer by having pap smears taken, despite already having had complete hysterectomies. Because these women no longer had their cervix, screening was unnecessary [14]. Every year, one million US children are submitted to unnecessary CT scans [15], the consequences of which are more than a mere waste of money: an estimated 29,000 cancers result from the approximately 70 million CT scans conducted in the US each year [16]. A representative study of 10,228 people from nine European countries revealed that 89% of men and 92% of women were not able to provide an estimate of the benefit of PSA testing and mammography screening or, if they did provide one, overestimated it by factors of ten, one hundred, and more [17]. Most doctors cannot evaluate the evidence for or against any specific treatment, nor can they critically judge reports in medical journals [17].

Patients must be protected from physicians who are unable to correctly interpret results from scientific investigations within the framework of evidence-based medicine and who fail to translate this interpretation into a therapeutic approach suited to their patients.

Example: a recently published international study of the value of PSA screening for prostate cancer found that it reduces the chance of dying from prostate cancer by 20% [18]. But how large a number is 20%, and to how many people does it correspond? Out of every 1,410 men who took part in regular screening, there was one less death of prostate cancer than in the equally large control group [19]. Sharing the burden has been advocated as an appropriate approach to involve patients in the decision making process. Since the late 1990s, when several publications on conceptual definitions of shared decision making emerged, interest in this approach has steadily grown [20]. In such shared processes, clinicians and patients, when faced with the task of making decisions, communicate together using the best evidence available [21]. This idea has been generally applied to patient-physician relationships as one of the defining features of the new professionalism in medicine [22]. The four main characteristics of shared decision making are:

1. both patient and physician are involved
2. both parties share information
3. both parties take steps to reach consensus on the preferred treatment
4. patient and physician reach agreement on which treatment to implement [23].

Early studies of cancer patients show that more than 60% expressed a desire to participate in clinical decisions [24, 25]. Patients want to know what is wrong, how the disease is called, whether it is serious enough to require expensive professional care, which alternative treatments exist, and how they can best cope with their situation. Physician-patient communication involves two aspects of medical care: the technical aspect, which is concerned with establishing a proper diagnosis and prescribing appropriate therapy, and the humanitarian aspect (the "good Samaritan" role), which involves supportive care. In the US, as well as in Europe, physician-patient communication is governed by the doctrine of informed consent, which has a determining influence on both the legal and ethical regulation of American and European medicine. It may be legally defined as the procedure whereby patients consent to or refuse medical intervention, based upon information provided by a healthcare professional, with regard to nature and potential consequences of any proposed intervention [26]. The ethical underpinnings of informed consent are self-determination and promotion of personal well-being. Failure to obtain informed consent constitutes a physician's refusal to respect the patient's autonomy. The three essential ingredients of autonomy are the ability to understand symptoms and outline necessary therapeutical steps, to make rational choices, and to appropriately act on these choices [9]. In order to act autonomously, "consumers" must first gain a reasonable level of understanding through education, information, and explanation [27]. The President's Commission for the Study of Ethical Problems in Medicine recognized shared decision making as an appropriate ideal for patient-professional relationships, which must be provided by any sound informed consent doctrine. "Ethically valid consent," the commission noted, "is a process of shared decision making based upon mutual respect and participation, not a ritual to be equated with reciting the contents of a form that details the risks of particular treatments" [28]. The doctrine of informed consent was stated succinctly by the Supreme Court of California, in the case of Cobbs v. Grant, as: "the patient's interest in information does not extend to a lengthy polysyllabic disclosure on all possible complications. A mini-course in medical science is not required; the patient is concerned with the risk of death or bodily harm and the problems of recuperation" [29]. Evidence suggests that a proper informed consent process directly impacts the quality of healthcare services [30–32]. Greenfield et al. [33] conclude that the interpersonal aspect of the physician-patient interaction may have an appreciable influence on a patient's outcome: they compared patients who were educated prior to surgery with those who were not and found a distinct improvement in outcome for the experimental group over the control group. A well-informed patient has a greater sense of control and is more likely to adhere to treatment. Since only patients that suffered poor outcome file malpractice suits, the value of the informed consent process in reducing malpractice losses may be undermined by a tendency to regard it as a means to protect the surgeon, rather than to educate the patient [34, 35]. For this reason, Brenner et al. [36] called for a new paradigm towards implementations of informed consent. This paradigm may embrace patient education and should abandon variants generated by attorneys whose sole aim is to absolve surgeons of liability exposure. There is no need to confront a well-educated patient with an exhaustive list of every conceivable complication. Rather, an educated patient must actively participate in a dialogue about the risks inherent in the planned surgery that are of importance to the individual decision-making process. Informed consent, shared decision making, and autonomy are hallmarks of quality in the 21st century, patient-centered medicine, in which the patient's subjective experience, values, and his full biographical background must be factored in. According to the Institute of Medicine, patient-centered-medicine is the basis of high-quality medical care [37, 38].

Patient-oriented medicine revolves around individual factors. In contrast, as one study showed, patients have an average 22 seconds to describe their symptoms, before being interrupted by the physician, who fears a lengthy discourse [39].

Drug therapy is an optimal treatment for patients with stable angina pectoris. Nevertheless, in the USA, in 2004, more than 1 million coronary stents were placed, 85% of which in cases of stable angina [40]. This is another example of non-patient-oriented medicine. Both in the USA and in Europe, exhaustive patient counseling and adequate drug treatment deliver less financial gains. However, the aim of therapeutic counseling should not be to overload the patient with an unmanageable amount of information but to provide real, usable knowledge about the disease and about the mechanism of action and possible side effects of any medications used. For this, the vast amount of side effects listed in package inserts, co-written by lawyers, is not important. As always, the physician must rather practice his traditional art of mitigating patients' fears and instill confidence in the course of treatment mutually agreed upon. It is not surprising that only ca. 57% of patients discharged from hospital after a coronary infarction said they understood the purpose of their prescribed medication [41]. Nor is it surprising that ca. 50% of drugs prescribed for chronic diseases is not taken by the patient [42]. Regardless of the climate created by contemporary high-performance medicine, with its basis in the natural sciences and modern technology, patients seek a sympathetic ear who, in their perception, doesn't see them as a disease process, but as an individual person. A substantial amount of fibromyalgia patients turn their back to technologized medicine and seek solace in so-called alternative medicine.

Successful therapeutic intervention requires mutual trust, nurtured by effective communication. A new physician-patient alliance, based on cooperation rather than confrontation, must be universally adopted. Physicians must accept their responsibility to be technical experts as well as for playing a supportive, interpersonal role. The polarization produced by the conflict between medical paternalism and patient sovereignty is counter-productive [9]. Patient safety advocates emphasize the importance of transparency with respect to medical errors. One way in which physicians may respond to an error is by apologizing – formally acknowledging the error and its consequences, taking responsibility, and expressing regret for causing harm – which may decrease blame and anger, increase trust, and improve patient-physician relationships. Apologies also have an important potential for decreasing the risk of a medical malpractice lawsuit and may help settle patient claims. Patients demand and expect explanations and apologies after medical errors [43]. Ethical standards, articulated by the American College of Physicians and the American Medical Association, require disclosure of errors. The Joint Commission, as well as many US states, requires hospitals and physicians to disclose adverse events to patients [44, 45]. In Germany, there are so far no federal regulations requiring physicians to disclose medical errors to their patients. As long as he does not stray from the facts, a physician may deny culpable wrongdoing. However, if it involves mitigating damage to the patient's health or preventing further damage, a physician must disclose complications that arise from treatment, without being asked to do so. A physician's duty to protect patients from harm being done to their health especially justifies mandatory disclosure when a complication or an error results in future treatment or surgery being necessary. In the opinion of the German Supreme Court, e.g., a physician involved in aftercare is required to point out obvious medical errors to his patients, because exposure to danger cannot be ethically justified [46]. A physician is also required to truthfully answer questions as to whether medical intervention has met generally accepted standards. However, a physician is not required to comment on possible reasons for deviating from the standard, because those reasons may substantiate malpractice claims [47]. A physician has a duty to truthfully state the facts. This is however not the same as admitting guilt. Under German law, a physician is required to obtain permission from his liability insurance company before pleading guilty, because, by prematurely doing so, he may lose coverage. This regulation is based on the view that it is a liability insurer's task to vouchsafe proper settlement of liability cases. However, in German case law, voices may be heard, pleading to make full disclosure a general requirement [48]. These voices are opposed by the common legal principle that nobody may be forced to indict himself and thereby expose himself to criminal prosecution. Similar to Germany or Europe, the USA has seen a rapidly increasing number of critically intensifying malpractice claims and lawsuits. Studdert et al. [49] cite a "deep seated tension between the malpractice system and the goals and initiatives of the patient-safety movement". Transparency with regard to matters of disclosure and reporting is a key initiative. In order to correct errors, one must be free to frankly and openly discuss them with all care providers working within the system. Thus, key patient safety proponents emphasize the importance of openness with respect to errors [50–52]. In contrast, tort systems in the USA and Europe target individual physicians and organizations and, due to the central role of negligence in matters of patient safety, focus on blame, punishment, and compensation. This system encourages secrecy and denial [53]. Open discussion of errors, complications, and patient death did not appear to lead to an increased risk of lawsuits. Out of 20,479 trauma-patients in Texas, 858 died. There were 4,301 ICU admissions and an estimated 5,367 cases of complications arising from treatment. From 1996 to 2004, the trauma department conducted weekly morbidity and mortality (M+M) conferences, open to any healthcare provider, including students, paramedics, nurses, allied health professionals, midlevel providers, resident physicians, and faculty physicians. The conference was advertised in the institutional newsletter and all deaths, major complications, and other adverse events were discussed. Only 7 patients filed a lawsuit [53].

The authors of the study came to the following conclusion: there is no medical-legal justification for secrecy and non-openness in processes aimed at performance improvement. An inclusive, multi-disciplinary M+M conference is an accepted forum for accurately and openly discussing errors and complications. Polk, in his address to the American Surgical Association, defined transparency as a "nothing to hide" approach, established through honest and open assessment within an organization, which aims to gain trust, improve collaboration, and maintain a higher level of credibility [54]. One of the most determined voices in support of transparency has been Leape's [55–58]. He cites three reasons why physicians are not inclined to report errors and adverse events: fear, lack of belief that reporting leads to improvement, and the time required to file a report. Studdert [59] raised a theoretical argument against disclosure, but there is limited empirical evidence on the topic [60]. Mazor found a protective effect of disclosure, in that he found the number of cases in which legal advice was sought to have decreased by 7.1% [61]. Schwappach [62] notes that in cases of severe adverse outcome, an honest, emphatic, and accountable approach decreased patients' support of strong sanctions for physicians by 59%. The ethical imperative should compel full disclosure to patients who have suffered preventable harm. Full disclosure may strengthen the patient-physician relationship and may reduce the desire to subject physicians to punitive measures. Gallagher [63, 64] and colleagues suggest "the norms, values, and practices that constitute the culture of medicine" may play a greater role in encouraging or inhibiting disclosure and apologies than does the risk of liability. Apologizing is difficult. Acknowledging an error conflicts with the quest for perfection and may result in a sense of vulnerability [65]. Finally, lack of certainty and skill in disclosing errors and in how to properly formulate an apology may prevent physicians from engaging in such conversations. Many of them have not been trained in how to effectively communicate with patients and, in particular, how to apologize after committing a medical error [66].

We must also keep in mind the suffering a physician is subjected to after committing a medical error. On the basis of their education and professional experience, physicians are expected to be able to cope with stressful and extreme situations in the increasingly complex world of modern medicine. After committing an error, a physician feels himself to be the second victim [67]. Self-doubt, feelings of guilt, and fear of failure develop, which may have long-term consequences such as depression, burnout, and loss of empathy.

An open safety culture makes it possible for a physician to not only admit the error to the patient, but most of all, it enables him to enter into dialogue with colleagues and superiors. Only then, that what happened may be further analyzed and the focus can shift from determining individual culpability to discovering and remedying systemic issues.

References

[1] Bourey, L, Martiny, M. Hippokrates und die griechische Medizin des klassischen Zeitalters. In: R. Toellner, Über die Epidemien I, 1986; p. 11.

[2] Kant, I, Kritik der praktischen Vernunft, I § 8.

[3] Beauchamp, TL, Childress, JF. Principles of Biomedical Ethics. 6th ed. Oxford Univ Press, Oxford.

[4] Freidson, E. Profession of Medicine: A Study in the sociology of applied knowledge. NY: Harper and Row, 1970; New York.

[5] Schneller, ES, Wilson, NA. Professionalism in 21th Century Professional Practice: Autonomy and Accountability in Orthopaedic Surgery Clin Orthop Relat. Res. 2009 October; 467(10):2561–2569.

[6] Eisenberg, L. The search of care: In: Knowles, JH (ed). Doing better and feeling worse. New York: Norton, 1977; 235–45.

[7] Burnum, JF. La maladie du petit papier: is writing a list of symptoms a sign of an emotional disorder? N Eng J Med 1985 Sep 12; 313(11):690–1. In: Rees, AM. Communication in the physician-patient relationship. Bull Med. Libr Assoc, 1993 January; 81(1).

[8] O'Dowd, TC. Five years of heartsink patients in general practice. BMJ 1988 Aug 20–27; 297:528–30.

[9] Rees, AM. Communication in the physician-patient relationship. Bull Med. Libr Assoc, 1993 January; 81(1).

[10] Katz, J. The silent world of doctor and patient. New York: Macmillan, 1982.

[11] Gigerenzer, G, Brighton, H. Homo heuristicus: why biased minds make better inferences. Top Cogn Sci 2009; 1:107–143.

[12] Gigerenzer, G, Gray, JAM. Better Doctors, Better Patients, Better Decisions. Envisioning Health Care 2020. The MIT Press, Cambridge, Massachusetts, London, England 2011; p 26–27.

[13] Adams, J. 2000/1765. The Revolutionary Writings of John Adams. Indianapolis; Liberty Fund. [1].

[14] Sivovich, B, Welch, H. Cervical cancer screening among women without a cervix. JAMA 2004; 291:2990–2993.

[15] Brenner, DJ, Hall, EJ. Computed tomography: An increasing source of radiation exposure. N Engl J Med 2007; 357:2277–2284.

[16] Gonzalez, AB, Mahesh, M, Kim, KP. et al.: Projected cancer risks from computed tomographic scans performed in the United States in 2007. Arch Intern Med 2009; 169(22):2071–2077.

[17] Gigerenzer, G. Gut feelings: The Intelligence of the Unconscious. New York 2007; Viking Press.

[18] Wilde, J. PSA screening cuts deaths by 20%, says world's largest prostate cancer study. ERSPC Press Office 2009; Carver Wilde Communications.

[19] Schröder, FH, Hugosson, J, Roobol, MJ. et al.: Screening and prostate-cancer mortality in a randomized European Study. N Engl J Med 2009; 360(13):1320–1328.

[20] Charles, CA, Gafni, A, Whelan, T. Shared decision-making in the medical encounter: What does it mean? Soc Sci Med 1997; 44:681–692.

[21] A. Coulter: Partnership with patients: To pros and cons of shared clinical decision making. J Health. Serv. Res. Policy 1997; 2:112–121.

[22] Schneller, ES, Wilson, NA. Professionalism in 21th century Professional Practice: Autonomy and Accountability in Orthopedic Surgery. Clin Orthop Relat Res 2009 October; 467(10):2561–2569.

[23] Stevenson, FA, Barry, CA, Britten, N, Barber, N, Bradley, CP. Doctor-patient communication about drugs: the evidence for shared decision making. Soc Sci Med. 2000; 50:829–840. [PubMed].

[24] Cassileth, B, Zupkis, R, Sutton-Smith, K. et al.: Information and participation preferences among cancer patients. Ann. Int. Med. 1980; 92:832–836.

[25] Blanchard, C, Labrecque, M, Ruckdeschel, J. et al.: Information and decision making preferences of hospitalized adult cancer patients. Soc. Sci. Med. 1988; 27:1139–1145.

[26] Annas, GJ. The rights of patients: the basic ACLU guide to patient rights. 2nd ed. Carbondale, IL: Southern Illinois Press, 1989; 83–4.

[27] Seedhouse, D. Liberating medicine. Chichester: Wiley, 1991; 119.

[28] President's Commission for the Study of Ethical Problems in Medicine and Biomedical Research. The ethical and legal implications of informed consent in the patient-practitioner relationship. Volume one: report: Washington, DC: U.S. Government Printing Office, 1982.

[29] Cobbs v. Grant 8 Cal. 2nd 229 (1972).

[30] Brody, DS, Miller, SM, Lerman, CE, Smith, DG, Caputo, GO. Patient perception of involvement in medical care: relationship to illness attitudes and outcomes. J Gen Intern Med. 1989; 4:506–611. [PubMed].

[31] Brody, DS, Miller, SM, Lerman, CE, Smith, DB, Lazaro, CG, Blum, MJ. The relationship between patient's satisfaction with their physicians and perceptions about interventions they desired and received. Med Care 1989; 27:1027–1035. [PubMed].

[32] Frosch, DL, Kaplan, RM. Shared decision making in clinical medicine: Past research and future directions. Am J Prev Med. 1999; 17:285–294. [PubMed].

[33] Greenfield, S, Kaplan, S, Ware, Jr, JE. Expanding patient involvement in care. Effects on patient outcomes. Ann Intern Med. 1985; 102:520–528 [PubMed].

[34] Ali, V. Consent forms as part of the informed consent process: Moving away from "medical Miranda". Hastings Law J. 2003; 54:1575–1591. [PubMed].

[35] Weithorn, LA, Scherer, DG. Children's involvement in research participation decisions: psychological considerations. In: Grodin, MA, Glantz, LH. eds. Children as Research Subjects. New York, NY: Oxford Press. 1994; 133–180.

[36] Brenner, LH, Brenner, AT, Horowitz, D. Beyond informed consent: Educating the Patient. Clin Orthop Relat Res. 2009 February; 467(2): 348–351.

[37] Epstein, RM, Peters, E. Beyond information. Exploring patient's preferences. JAMA 2009; 302:195–197.

[38] Kreß, H. Medizinische Ethik. Gesundheitsschutz – Selbstbestimmungsrechte – Heutige Wertkonflikte. 2nd ed. Stuttgart, Kohlhammer, 2009.

[39] Langwitz, W, Denz, M, Keller, A. et al.: Spontaneous talking time at start of consultation in outpatient clinic. BMJ 2002; 325:682–683.

[40] Boden, WE, O'Rourke, RA, Teo, K. et al.: Optimal medical therapy with or without PCI for stable coronary disease. N Engl J Med 2007; 356:1503–1516.

[41] Calkins, DR, Davis, RB, Reiley, P. et al.: Patient-physician communication at hospital discharge and patient's understanding of the postdischarge treatment plan. Arch. Intern Med 1997; 157:1026–1030.

[42] Marinker, M, Shaw, J. Not to be taken as directed. BMJ 2003; 326:348–349.

[43] Robbennolt, JK. Apologies and Medical Error. Clin Orthop Relat Res. 2009 February; 467(2):376–382.

[44] Gallagher, TH, Studdert, D, Levinson, W. Disclosing harmful medical errors to patients. N Engl J Med 2007; 356:2713–2719. Joint Commission on the Accreditation of Healthcare Organization. Hospital Accreditation Standards. Standard RI.2.90 OAK Brook, IL: Joint Commission Resources; 2005.

[45] Robbennolt, JK. Apologies and settlement levers. J Empir Legal Studies. 2006; 3:333–373.

[46] Weltrich, H. Offenbarungspflicht bei ärztlichen Behandlungsfehlern? Gynäkologe 2004; 37:277–278.

[47] BGH, NJW 1984; p. 661.

[48] NJW 2000; p. 1749.

[49] Studdert, DM, Mello, MM, Brennan, TA. Medical malpractice. N Engl J Med 2004; 350: 283–290. [PubMed].

[50] Lo, B. Resolving Ethical Dilemmas: A Guide for Clinicians, 2nd ed. Lippincott: Williams and Wilkins, Philadelphia, 2000.

[51] Witman, AB, Park, DM, Hardin, SB. How do patients want physicians to handle mistakes? A survey of internal medicine patients in an academic setting. Arch Intern Med. 1996; 156(22): 2565–9.

[52] Wu, AW, Cavanaugh, TA, McPhee, SJ, Lo, B, Micco, GP. To tell the truth: ethical and practical issues in disclosing medical mistakes to patients. J Gen Intern Med 1997; 12(12):770–5. [PMC free article].

[53] Stewart, RM, Corneille, MG, Johnston, JJ. et al.: Transparent and open Discussion of Errors does not increase Malpractice Risk in Trauma Patients. Ann Surg 2006 May; 243(5): 645–651.

[54] Polk, HC. Quality, safety and transparency. Ann Surg 2005; 242:293–301. [PMC free article] [PubMed].

[55] Leape, LL. Why should we report adverse incidents? J Eval Clin Pract. 1999; 5:1–4. [PubMed].

[56] Leape, LL. Reporting of adverse events. N Engl J Med. 2002; 347:1633–1639. [PubMed].

[57] Leape, LL. Reporting of medical errors: time for a reality check. Qual Safety Healthcare. 2000; 9:144–145.

[58] Leape, LL. Making health care safe: are we up to it? J Pediatr Surg. 2004; 39:258–268. [PubMed].

[59] Studdert, DM, Mello, MM, Gawande, AA, Brennan, TA, Wang, YC. Disclosure of medical injury to patients: an improbable risk management strategy. Health Aff (Millwood). 2007; 26(1):215–26. [PubMed].

[60] Wu, AW, Huang, JCh, Stokes, S. et al. Disclosing Medical Errors to Patients: It's not what you say, it's what they hear. J Gen Int Med. 2009 September; 24(9):1012–1017.

[61] Mazor, KM, Reed, GW, Yood, RA, Fischer, MA, Baril, J, Gurwitz, JW. Disclosure of medical errors: what factors influence how patients respond? J Gen Intern Med 2006; 21(7):704–10.

[62] Schwappach, DL, Koeck, CM. What makes an error unacceptable? A factorial survey on the disclosure of medical errors. Int J Qual Health Care. 2004; 16(4):317–26. [PubMed].

[63] Gallagher, TH, Waterman, AD, Ebers, AG, Fraser, VJ, Levinson, W. Patient's and physicians' attitudes regarding the disclosure of medical errors. JAMA. 2003; 289:1001–1007. [PubMed].

[64] Gallagher, TH, Waterman, AD, Garbutt, JM, Kapp, JM, Chan, DK, Dunagan, WC, Fraser, VJ, Levinson. W. US and Canadian physicians' attitudes and experience regarding disclosing errors to patients. Arch Intern Med. 2006; 166:1605–1611. [PubMed].

[65] Kaldjian, LC, Jones, EW, Rosenthal, GE, Tripp-Reimer, T, Hillis, SL. An empirically derived taxonomy of factors affecting physicians' willingness to disclose medical errors. J Gen Intern Med. 2006; 21:942–948. [PMC free article] [PubMed].

[66] Full Disclosure Working Group, Harvard University. When things go wrong: responding to adverse events. March 2006. Available at: www.macoalition.org/documents/respondingToAdverseEvents.pdf. Accessed August 14, 2008.

[67] Wu, AW. Medical error: the second victim. The doctor who makes the mistakes needs help too. BMJ 2000; 320:726.

Bibliography

Adams, J. 2000/1765. The Revolutionary Writings of John Adams. Indianapolis; Liberty Fund. [1].

Adamsen, S, Hansen, OH, Funch-Jensen, P. et al. Bile duct injury during laparoscopic cholecystectomy. A prospective nationwide series. J Am Coll Surg 1997; 184:571.

Addiss, DG, Shaffer, N, Fowler, BS. et al. The epidemiology of appendicitis and appendectomy in the United States. Am J Epidemiol 1990; 132:910–925.

AHCA. Florida Agency for Healthcare Administration Web site. 2003. http://www.fdhc.state.fl.us/. Accessed June 18, 2006.

Ahrendt, GM, Gardner, K, Barbul, A. Loss of colonic structural collagen impairs healing during intra-abdominal sepsis. Arch Surg 1994; 129:1179.

Akerström, G, Malmaeus, J, Bergstrom, R. Surgical anatomy of human parathyroid glands. Surgery 1984; 95:14.

Aktionsbündnis Patientensicherheit: Agenda Patientensicherheit 2007, Witten 2007.

Aleccia, J. MSNBC Health Care. Medical litter: device debris poses serious risk. Available online at: http://msnbc.msn.com/id/25120613/. Last accessed on July 28, 2008.

Ali, V. Consent forms as part of the informed consent process: Moving away from "medical Miranda". Hastings Law J. 2003; 54:1575–1591. [PubMed].

Al-Kubati, WR. Bile duct injury following laparoscopic cholecystectomy. A Clinical Study Saudi J Gastroenterol. 2010 April; 16 (2), 100–104.

Al-Saeed, AH. Medical Liability litigation in Saudi-Arabia. Saudi J Anaesth 2010 Sep–Dec; 4 (3):122–126.

Alves, A, Panis, Y, Trancart, D, Regimbeau, JM, Pocard, M, Valleur, P. Factors associated with clinically significant anastomotic leakage after large bowel resection: multivariate analysis of 707 patients. World J Surg 2002; 26:499.

American Academy of Ophthalmology. Minimizing wrong IOL placement: patient safety bulletin number 2. AAO Web site. http://www.aao.org/aao/education/library/safety/iol.cfm. Accessed November 28, 2005.

Amid, PK, Shulman, AG, Lichtenstein, EL. Die Herniotomie nach Lichtenstein. Chirurg 1994; 65:54.

Amid, PK, Shulman, AG, Lichtenstein, IL. Critical scrutiny of the open tension-free hernioplasty. Am J Surg 1993; 165:369.

Anderson, PE, Hurley, PR, Rosswick, P. Conservative treatment and long term prophylactic thyroxine in the prevention of recurrence of multinodular goiter. Surg Gynecol Obstet 1990; 171:309.

Andersson, RE, Hugander, A, Thulin, AJG. Diagnostic accuracy and perforation rate in appendicitis: association with age and sex of the patient and with appendectomy rate. Eur J Surg 1992; 158:37–41.

Ando, N, Ozawa, S, Kitagawa, Y, Shinozawa, Y, Kitajima, M. Improvement in the results of surgical treatment of advanced squamous esophageal carcinoma during 15 consecutive years. Ann Surg 2000; 232:225–32.

Annas, GJ. The rights of patients: the basic ACLU guide to patient rights. 2nd ed. Carbondale, IL: Southern Illinois Press, 1989; 83–4.

Apter, S, Hertz, M, Rubinstein, ZJ, Zissin, R. Gossypiboma in the early post-operative period: a diagnostic problem. Clin Radiol 1990; 42(2):128.

Archibold, RC. Girl in transplant mix-up dies after two weeks. New York Times. February 23, 2003; 1:18.

Ashton, P, Kuhn, R, Collopy, B. Small bowel incarceration after laparoscopically assisted vaginal hysterectomy – a preventable complication? Aust N Z J Obstet Gynaecol 1995; 35:352.

Associated Press. Hospital pulls plug on the wrong patient. Toronto Star. March 13, 1995; A.2.

Babcock, JR, McKinley, WM. Acute appendicitis: an analysis of 1,662 consecutive cases. Ann Surg 1959; 150:131–141.

Baer, M, van Dyck, C, Frese, M. et al. Organizational Errors Management Culture and its Impact on Performance: A two-study-Replication, In: Journal of Applied Psychology 2005; Vol 90, no 6, p 1228–1240.

Baker, GR, Norton, PG, Flintoft, V. et al. The Canadian adverse events study: the incidence of adverse events study: the incidence of adverse events among hospital patients in Canada. CMAJ 2004; 170:1678–1186.

Bal, Sonny, B. An Introduction to the Medical Malpractice in the United States. In: Clin Orthop Relat Res. 2009; 467 (2):339–347.

Ballem, RV, Rudomanski, J. Techniques of Pneumoperitoneum. Surg Laparosc Endosc 1993; 3:42.

Bani-Hani, KE, Gharaibeh, KA, Yaghan, RJ. Retained surgical sponges (gossypiboma). Asian J Surg 2005; 28:109–115.

Barach, P, Small, SD. Reporting and preventing medical mishaps: lessons from non-medical near miss reporting systems. BMJ 2000; 320:759–763.

Barkan, H, Webster, S, Ozeran, S. Factors predicting the recurrence of adhesive small bowel obstruction. Am J Surg. 1995; 170:361–365.

Barnett, WO, Petro, AB, Williamson, JW A current appraisal of problems with gangrenous bowel. Ann Surg 1976; 183:653.

Bartels, H, Barthlen, W, Siewert, JR. The therapeutic results of programmed relaparotomy in diffuse peritonitis. Chirurg 1992; 63:174–180.

Bartels, H. Spezielle Gesichtspunkte postoperativer Komplikationen in der Viszeralchirurgie. Chirurg 2009; 80:780–789.

Barth, U. Vorkommnismeldungen bei Klammernahtinstrumenten. Chirurg 2009; 80:735–740.

Bassini, E. Über die Behandlung des Leistenbruches. Arch Klin Chir 1890; 40:429.

Bates, DW, Cullen, DJ, Laird, N. et al. ADE Prevention Study Group. Incidence of adverse drug events and potential adverse drug events: Implications for prevention. JAMA. 1995; 274: 29–34.

Bauch, J, Bruch, HP, Heberer, J, Jähne, J. Behandlungsfehler und Haftpflicht in der Viszeralchirurgie. Springer Verlag Heideberg, 2011.

Beard, JD, Nicholson, ML, Sayers, RD, Lloyd, D, Everson, NW. Intraoperative air testing of colorectal anastomoses: a prospective randomized trial. Br J Surg 1990; 77(10):1095–1097.

Beauchamp, TL, Childress, JF. Principles of Biomedical Ethics. 6th ed. Oxford Univ Press, Oxford.

Becker, K, Hofler, H. Pathophysiologie der Appendizitis. Chirurg 2002; 73:777–781.

Becker, WF. Acute adhesive ileus. A study of 412 cases with particular reference to the abuse of tube decompression in treatment. Surg. Gynecol. Obstet 1952; 95:472.

Bellomo, R, Goldsmith, D, Uchino S. et al. Prospective controlled trial of effect of medical emergency team on postoperative morbidity and mortality rates. Crit Care 2004; 32:916–921.

Below, KH. Der Arzt im Römischen Recht. In: Münchner Beiträge zur Papyrusforschung und antiken Rechtsgeschichte. München: Beck'sche Verlagsbuchhandlung, 1953.

Ben-David, K, Rossidis, G, Zlotecki, RA. et al. Minimally invasive esophagectomy is safe and effective following neoadjuvant chemoradiation therapy. Ann Surg Oncol 2011; 18:3324–3329.

Bergamaschi, R, Becouam, G, Ronceray, J, Arnaud, JP. Morbidity of thyroid surgery. Am J Surg 1998; 176:71–75.

Berger, C, Hartmann, M, Wildemann, B. Progressive visual loss due to a muslinoma – report of a case and review of the literature. Eur J Neurol 2003; 10:153–158.

Bergman, JJ, van den Brink, GR, Rauws, EA, de Wit, L, Obertop, H, Huibregtse, K. et al. Treatment of bile duct lesions after laparoscopic cholecystectomy. Gut 1996; 38:141–147.

Berkowitz, S, Marshall, H, Charles, A. Retained intra-abdominal surgical instruments: time to use nascent technology? Am Surg 2007; 73:1083–1085.

Berner. Anzahl von Begutachtungen im Rahmen der Behandlung eines Gallensteinleidens. Personal communication, German Medical Association 2009; Berlin.

Berry, J, Malt, RA. Appendicitis near its centenary. Ann Surg 1984; 200:567–575.

Betz, RP, Levy, HB. An interdisciplinary method of classifying and monitoring medication errors. Am J Hosp Pharm 1985; 42:1724–1732.

Beyea, S. Counting instruments and sponges. AORN J 2003; 78:290–292.

BGH, NJW 1984; p. 661.

BGH, Urteil v. 27.11.1981 – VIZR 138/79.

BGH, VersR 1953, 338; VersR 1964, 392; VersR 1955, 344.

Bhasale, AL, Miller, GC, Reid, S, Britt, HC. Analysing potential harm in Australian general practice; an incident-monitoring study. Med J Aust 1998; 169:73–6.

Bhatti, CS, Tamijmarane, A, Bramhall, SR. A tale of three spilled gallstones: one liver mass and two abscesses. Dig Surg 2006; 23:198–200.

Bhoyrul, S, Payne J, Steffens, B. et al. A randomized prospective study of radially expanding trocars in laparoscopic surgery. J Gastrointest Surg 2000; 4:302–397.

Bhoyrul, S, Payne, J, Steffens, B, Swanstrom, L, Way, LW. A randomized prospective study of radially expanding trocars in laparoscopic surgery. J Gastrointest Surg 4:392.

Biondo, S, Parés, D, Kreisler, E. et al. Anastomotic dehiscence after resection and primary anastomoses in left-sided colonic emergencies. Dis Colon Rectum 2005; 48(12):2272–2280.

Bismuth, H, Lazorthes, F. Les traumatismes opératoires de la voie biliaire principale. 1982; Masson, Paris.

Bittner, R, Kraft, K, Schwarz, J, Leibl, B. Risiko und Nutzen der Laparoskopischen Hernioplastik (TAPP), 5 Jahre Erfahrungen bei 3,400 Hernienreparationen. Chirurg 1998; 69:854.

Bjorck, M. et al. Die akute mesenteriale Ischämie. Chirurg 2003; 74:419–431.

Blanchard, C, Labrecque, M, Ruckdeschel, J. et al.: Information and decision making preferences of hospitalized adult cancer patients. Soc. Sci. Med. 1988; 27:1139–1145.

Blumgart, LH, Kelley, CJ, Benjamin, IS. Benign bile duct stricture following cholecystectomy: critical factors in management. Br J Surg 1984; 71:836.

Boden, WE, O'Rourke, RA, Teo, K. et al.: Optimal medical therapy with or without PCI for stable coronary disease. N Engl J Med 2007; 356:1503–1516.

Böhm, B, Schwenk, W, Junghans, T. Das Pneumoperitoneum, Auswirkungen der Laparoskopie auf die Organsysteme. 2000; Springer-Verlag.

Boike, GM, Miller, CE, Spirtos, NM. et al. Incisional bowel herniations after operative laparoscopy: a series of nineteen cases and review of the literature. Am J Obstet Gynecol 1995; 6:1726.

Boley, SJ, Feinstein, FR, Sammartano, R. et al. New concepts in the management of emboli of the superior mesenteric artery. Surg Gynecol Obstet 1981; 153:561–9.

Bonjer, HJ, Hazebroek, EJ, Kazemier, G. et al. Open versus closed establishment of Pneumoperitoneum in laparoscopic surgery. Br J Surg. 1997; 84:599.

Bononi, M, de Cesare, A, Atella, F. et al. Surgical treatment of multinodular goiter: incidence of lesions of the recurrent nerves after total thyroidectomy. Int Surg 2000; 85:190–193.

Bosma, E, Veen, EJ, Roukema, JA. Incidence, nature and impact of error in surgery. Br J Surg. 2011; June 27.

Bosscha, K, Hulstaert, PF, Visser, MR., van Vroonhoven, ThJMV, van der Werken, Chr. Open management of the abdomen and planned reoperations, in severe bacterial peritonitis. Eur J Surg 2000; 166:44–49.

Bourey, L, Martiny, M. Hippokrates und die griechische Medizin des klassischen Zeitalters. In: R. Toellner, Über die Epidemien I, 1986; p. 11.

Bower, S, Moore, BB, Weiss, SM. Neuralgia after inguinal hernia repair. Am Surg 1996; 62: 664–7.

Bozzetti, F, Marubini, E, Bonfanti, G. et al. Total versus subtotal gastrectomy: Surgical morbidity and mortality rates in a multicenter Italian randomized trail. The Italian Gastrointestinal Tumor Study Group. Ann Surg 1997; 226:613–620.

Brennan, TA, Laird, MM. et al. The nature of adverse events and negligence in hospitalized patients. Results of the Harvard Medical Practice Study II. N Engl J Med 1991; 324:377–384.

Brennan, TA, Leape, LL, Laird, MM. et al. Incidence of adverse events and negligence in hospitalized patients. Results of the Harvard Medical Practice Study I. N Engl J Med 1991; 324:370–376.

Brenner, DJ, Hall, EJ. Computed tomography: An increasing source of radiation exposure. N Engl J Med 2007; 357:2277–2284.

Brenner, LH, Brenner, AT, Horowitz, D. Beyond informed consent: Educating the Patient. Clin Orthop Relat Res. 2009 February; 467(2): 348–351.

Breukink, S, Pierie, J, Wiggers, T. Laparoscopic versus open total mesorectal excision for rectal cancer. Cochrane Database Syst Rev 2006; CD005200.

Britten, N, Stevenson, FA, Barry, CA, Barber, N, Bradley, CP. Misunderstandings in prescribing decisions in general practice: qualitative study. BMJ 2000; 320:484–8.

Brody, DS, Miller, SM, Lerman, CE, Smith, DB, Lazaro, CG, Blum, MJ. The relationship between patient's satisfaction with their physicians and perceptions about interventions they desired and received. Med Care 1989; 27:1027–1035. [PubMed].

Brody, DS, Miller, SM, Lerman, CE, Smith, DG, Caputo, GO. Patient perception of involvement in medical care: relationship to illness attitudes and outcomes. J Gen Intern Med. 1989; 4:506–611. [PubMed].

Bruce, J, Krukowski, ZH, Al-Khairy, G. et al. Systematic review of the definition and measurement of anastomotic leak after gastrointestinal surgery. Br J Surg 2001; 88:1157–1168.

Bruch, HP. Ileus-Krankheit. Chirurg 1989; 60:198–202.

Brümmer, S, Sohr, D, Gastmeier, P. Intra-abdominal abscesses and laparoscopic versus open appendectomies. Infect Control Hosp Epidemiol 2009; 30:713–715.

Büchler, MW, Baer, HU, Brugger, LE. et al. Surgical therapy of diffuse peritonitis: debridement and intraoperative extensive lavage. Chirurg 1997; 68:811–815.

Budetti, P, Waters, TM. Medical Malpractice law in the United States. In: The Kaiser Family Foundation. 2005; p. 1–5.

Budetti, P, Waters, TM. Medical Malpractice law in the United States. In: The Henry J. Kaiser Family Foundation. 2005; http://www.kff.org.

Burnum, JF. La maladie du petit papier: is writing a list of symptoms a sign of an emotional disorder? N Eng J Med 1985 Sep 12; 313(11):690–1. In: Rees, AM. Communication in the physician-patient relationship. Bull Med. Libr Assoc, 1993 January; 81(1).

Büter, F. Inauguraldissertation "Sogenannte Kunstfehler" im Sektionsgut des Institutes für Rechtsmedizin in Hamburg (2002–2006) unter besonderer Berücksichtigung endoskopischer und laparoskopischer Eingriffe. Hamburg 2009.

Caldwell, CB, Ricotta, JJ. Changes in visceral blood flow with elevated intraabdominal pressure. J Surg Res 1987; 43:14–20.

Calkins, DR, Davis, RB, Reiley, P. et al.: Patient-physician communication at hospital discharge and patient's understanding of the postdischarge treatment plan. Arch. Intern Med 1997; 157: 1026–1030.

Callesen, T, Bech, K, Kehlet, H. Prospective study of chronic pain after groin hernia repair. Br J Surg 1999; 86:1528–1531.

Calvete, J, Sabater, L, Camps, B. et al: Bile duct injury during laparoscopic cholecystectomy: myth or reality of the learning curve? Surg Endosc. 2000; 14:608–611.

Calzavacca, P, Licari, E, Tee, A. et al. The impact of rapid response system on delayed emergency team activation patient characteristics and outcomes – a follow-up study. Resuscitation 2010; 81:31–35.

Canale, ST. Wrong-site surgery: a preventable complication. Clin Orthop Relat Res 2005; 433:26–29.

Carey. LC Cholecystectomy – a new standard. Ann Surg 1992; 216:617.

Carroll, BJ, Birth, M, Phillips, EH. Common bile duct injuries during laparoscopic cholecystectomy that result in litigation. Surg Endosc. 1998; 12:310–313. Discussion 314.

Carstensen, G. Chirurgie und Recht, In: Häring, R (ed). Chirurgie und Recht, Berlin 1983; p. 3–7.

Carty, NJ, Keating, J, Campbell, J, Karanjia, N, Heald, RJ. Prospective audit of an extramucosal technique for intestinal anastomoses. Br J Surg 1991; 78:1439.

Cassileth, B, Zupkis, R, Sutton-Smith, K. et al.: Information and participation preferences among cancer patients. Ann. Int. Med. 1980; 92:832–836.

Catarci, M, Carlini, M, Gentileschi, P. et al. Major and minor injuries during the creation of Pneumoperitoneum. A multicenter study on 12,919 cases. Surg Endosc. 2001; 15:566–569.

Chandler, JG, Voyles, CR, Floore, TH. et al. Litigious consequences of open and laparoscopic biliary surgical mishaps. J Gastrointest Surg. 1997; 1:138–145.

Chang, A, Schyve, PM, Croteau, RJ. et al. The JCAHO patient safety event taxonomy: a standardized terminology and classification schema for near misses and adverse events. International Journal for Quality in Health Care 2005; Vol 17, No 2: p 95–105.

Chapman, WC, Halevy, A, Blumgart, LH, Benjamin, IS. Postcholecystectomy bile duct strictures. Arch Surg 1995; 130:597.

Chaprou, C, Pierre, F, Querleu, D. et al. Major vascular complications from gynaecologic laparoscopy. Gynecol Obstet Fertil 2000; 28:880–887.

Charles, C, Gafni, A, Whelan, T. Shared decision-making in the medical encounter: what does it mean? (Or it takes at least two to tango). Soc Sci Med. 1997; 44:681–682.

Chasseray, VM, Kiroff, GK, Buard, JL, Launois, BL. Cervical on thoracic anastomoses for esophagectomy for carcinoma. Surg Gynec Obstetrics 1989; 169:55–62.

Chassin, MR, Becher, EC. The wrong patient. Ann Int Med 2002; 136:826–833.

Chiofalo, R, Holzinger, F, Klaiber, C. Total extraperitoneale Netzplastik bei primären und Rezidivhernien – Gibt es Unterschiede? Chirurg 2001; 72:1485.

Chlang, H. Mom awarded $ 1 million over embryo mix-up. San Francisco Chronicle. August 4, 2004; B 4. http://sfgate.com/cgi-bin/article.cgi?file=/chronicle/archive/2004/08/04/BAGN382-BII1.DTL. Accessed November 28, 2005.

Christof-Veit, JB, Döbler, K, Fischer, B. Qualität sichtbar machen. BQS-Qualitätsreport 2008. In: BQS Bundesgeschäftsstelle Qualitätssicherung GmbH, Düsseldorf, 2009; p. 52.

Christou, NV, Barie, PS, Dellinger, EP, Waymack, JP, Stone, HH. Surgical Infection Society intra-abdominal infection study. Prospective evaluation of management techniques and outcome. Arch Surg 1993; 128:193–198.

Clark, GWB, Peter, JH, Ireland, AP. et al. Nodal metastasis and sites of recurrence after en-bloc esophagectomy for adenocarcinoma. Ann Thorac Surg 1994; 58:646–654.

Clark, MA, Plamk, LD, Hill, GL. Wound healing associated with severe surgical illness. World J Surg 2000; 24:648.

Clark, OH. TSH suppression in the management of thyroid nodules and thyroid cancer. World J Surg 1981; 5:39.

Clavien, PA, Sanabria, JR, Mentha, G. et al. Recent results of elective open cholecystectomy in a North American and a European Center. Comparison of complications and risk factors. Ann Surg 1992; 216:618–626.

Clinical Outcomes of Surgical Therapy Study Group. A comparison of laparoscopically assisted and open colectomy for colon cancer. N Engl J Med 2004; 350(20):2050–2059.

Cobbs v. Grant 8 Cal. 2nd 229 (1972).

Conciliation Committee of the State Chamber of Medicine in Rhineland-Palatinate. Proceedings 003/07. Published 02.05.2008. "Ärzteblatt Rhineland-Pfalz", January 2011, Vol. 1, p. 17.

Connor, S, Garden, OJ. Bile duct injury in the era of laparoscopic cholecystectomy. Br J Surg. 2006; 93:158–68.

Coquelle, IJ, Cura, B, Fourest, B. Safety, Culture and Quality System. In: Carino, A, Weiman, G (ed). Proceedings of the International Topical Meeting on Safety Culture in Nuclear Installations; American Nuclear Society of Austria, Vienna, 1995; p 193–202.

Cougard, P, Osmak, L, Esquis, P. et al. Endoscopic thyroidectomy. A preliminary report including 40 patients. Ann Chir 2005; 130:81–85.

Coulter, A. Partnership with patients: To pros and cons of shared clinical decision making. J Health. Serv. Res. Policy 1997; 2:112–121.

Cowell, HR. Wrong-site surgery [editorial]. J Bone Joint Surg Am. 1998; 80:463.

Cox, MR, Gunn, IF, Eastman, MC et al. The operative aetiology and types of adhesions causing small bowel obstruction. Aust NZ J Surg 1993; 63:848–852.

Cox, MR, Gunn, JF, Eastman, MC et al. The safety and duration of non-operative treatment for adhesive small-bowel obstruction. Aust NZ J Surg. 1993; 63:367.

Cox, S, Cox, T. The structure of Employee Attitudes to Safety: An European Example. In: Work and Stress, 1991; Vol 5, No 2, p 189–201.

Cox, S, Flin, RF. Safety culture: Philosopher's Stone or Man of Straw? In: Work and Stress, 1998; Vol 12, No 3, p 189–201.

Crosby, PB. Qualitätsmanagement, 2000, Wien.

Csendes, A, Navarrete, C, Burdiles, P, Yarmuch, J. Treatment of common bile duct injuries during laparoscopic cholecystectomy: endoscopic and surgical management. World J Surg 2001; 25:1346–1351.

Cuschieri, A, Dubois, F, Mouret, P. et al. The European experience with laparoscopic cholecystectomy. Am J Surg 1991; 161: 385–387.

Davidoff, AM, Pappas, TN, Murray, EA. et al. Mechanism of major biliary injury during laparoscopic cholecystectomy. Am J Surg. 1992; 215:196–298.

Davids, PHP, Ringers, J, Rauws, EAJ, de Wit, LT. et al. Bile duct inury after laparoscopic cholecystectomy the value of endoscopic retrograde cholangiopancreaticography. Gut 1993; 34:1250.

Davis, P, Lay-Yee, R, Briant, R. et al. Preventable in-hospital medical injury under the "no fault" system in New Zealand. Qual Safe Health Care. 2003 August; 12 (4):251–256.

De Dombal, FT. Diagnosis of acute abdominal pain. Edinburgh, London, Melbourne, New York: Churchill Livingstone 1991.

De Dombal, FT. The OMGE acute abdominal pain survey. Progress report, 1986. Scand J Gastroenterol 1988; 23 (144):36–42.

De Reuver, PR, Dijkgraat, MG, Gevers, SK. et al. Poor agreement among expert witnesses in bile duct injury malpractice litigation: an expert panel survey. Ann Surg 2008; 248:815–820.

De Ville, KA. Medical Malpractice in Nineteenth Century America: Origins and legacy. New York, NY: NYU-Press; 1990.

Dekker, SW, Hugh, TB. Laparoscopic bile duct injury: understanding the psychology and heuristics of the error. ANZ J Surg 2008; 78:1109–1114.

Delbridge, L, Guinea, AL, Reeve, TS. Total thyroidectomy for bilateral benign multinodular goiter: effect of changing practice. Arch Surg 1999; 134:1389–1393.

Dellinger, RP. Cardiovascular management of septic shock. Crit Care Med. 2003; 31:946–55.

Deutsche Gesellschaft für Chirurgie. Leitlinien zur Therapie der benignen Struma – G80. Mitt. Deutsch Ges Chir 1998; 3.

DeVita, MA, Aulisio, MP. The ethics of medical mistakes: historical, legal, and institutional perspectives. Kennedy Inst. Ethics J. 2001; 11:115–116.

Deziel, DJ, Millikan, KW, Economou, SG. et al. Complications of laparoscopic cholecystectomy: a national survey of 4,292 hospitals and an analysis of 77,604 cases. Am J Surg. 1993; 165:9–14.

Di Giovanni, CW, Kang, L, Manuel, J. Patient compliance in avoiding wrong-site surgery. J Bone Joint Surg Am. 2003; 85-A:815–819.

Diller, H. Das Gesetz. In: Hippokrates. Ausgewählte Schriften. Philipp Reclam jun., Stuttgart, 1984; p. 120.

Dippolito, A, Braslow, BM, Lombardo, G. et al. How David beat Goliath: history of physicians fighting frivolous law suits. OPUS 12 Scientist 2008; 2(1):1–8.

Dixon, JM, Elton, RA, Reiney, JB. et al. DAD: Rectal examination in patients with pain in the right lower quadrant of the abdomen. BMJ 1990; 302:386–388.

Docherty, JG, Mc Gregor, JR, Akyol, AM, Murray, GD, Galloway, DJ. West of Scotland and Highland Anastomoses Study Group. Comparison of manually constructed and stapled anastomoses in colorectal surgery. Ann Surg 1995; 221(2):176–184.

Dolan, JP, Diggs, BS, Sheppard, BG, Hunter, JG. Ten-year trend in the national volume of bile duct injuries requiring operative repair. Surg Endosc. 2005; 19:967–973.

Dolgin, SE, Beck, AR, Tartter, PI. The risk of perforation when children with possible appendicitis are observed in the hospital. Surg Gynecol Obstet 1992; 175:320.

Dovey, SM, Meyers, DS, Phillips, RL, Jr. et al. A preliminary taxonomy of medical errors in family practice. Qual Saf Health Care 2002; 11:233–8.

Dralle, H, Pichlmayr, R. Risikominderung bei Rezidiveingriffen wegen benigner Struma. Chirurg 1991; 62:169.

Dralle, H, Scheumann, GEW, Hundeshagen, H. et al. Die transsternale zervikomediastinale Primärtumorresektion und Lymphadenektomie beim Schilddrüsenkarzinom. Langenbecks Arch Chir 377:34–44.

Dralle, H, Sekulla, C, Lorenz, K. et al. Intraoperative monitoring of the recurrent larnygeal nerve in thyroid surgery. World J Surg 2008; 32:1358–1366.

Dralle, H. Rekurrens- und Nebenschilddrüsenoperation in der Schilddrüsenchirurgie. Chirurg 2009; 80:352–363.

Dubois, F, Berthelot, G, Levard, H. [Laparoscopic cholecystectomy. Technique and complications. Report of 2,665 cases]. Bull Acad Natl Med 1995; 179:1059–1066; discussion 1066–1068.

Düllinger, F. Krankenhaus-Management im Spannungsfeld zwischen Patientenorientierung und Rationalisierung: Probleme und Gestaltungsmöglichkeiten des Business Reengineering in der Krankenhaus-Praxis, München 1996.

Dumont, JE, Lamy, F, Roger, P, Maenhaut, C. Physiological and pathological regulation of thyroid cell proliferation and differentiation by thyrotropin and other factors. Physiol. Rev 1992; 72:667.

Dunn, D. Surgical site verification: A through Z. J Perianesth Nurs. 2006; 21:317–331.

Dunn, DC, Watson, CJE. Disposable guarded trocar and cannular in laparoscopic surgery: a caveat Br J Surg. 1992; 79:927.

Dunn, EB, Wolfe, JJ. Medication error classification and avoidance. Hosp Pharm 1997; 32:860–865.

Eckes, G. The Six Sigma Revolution: How General Electric and Others Turned Process into Profits, 2001; New York.

Eckhart, WV. Geschichte der Medizin. Springer, Berlin-Heidelberg-New York, 1998.

Eckstein, HH. Die akute Mesenterialischämie. Chirurg 2003; 74:419–431.

Editorial British Medical Journal BMJ 320; 730; March 2000.

Egorova, NN, Moskowitz, A, Gelijns, A. et al. Managing the prevention of retained surgical instruments: what is the value of counting? Ann Surg 2008; 247:13–18.

Eisenberg, L. The search of care: In: Knowles, JH (ed). Doing better and feeling worse. New York: Norton, 1977; 235–45.

Elder, NC, Dovey, SM. Classification of medical errors and preventable adverse events in primary care: A synthesis of the literature. The Journal of Family Practice; November 2002, Vol. 51, No. 11.

Ellis, H, Moran, BJ, Thompson, JN. et al. Adhesion-related hospital readmissions after abdominal and pelvic surgery: a retrospective cohort study. Lancet 1999; 353:1476–1480.

Ellis, Jr. FH, Heatly, GJ, Krasna, MJ, Williamson, WA, Balogh, K. Esophagogastrectomy for carcinoma of the esophagus and cardia: a comparison of findings and results after standard resection in three consecutive eight-year intervals with improved staging criterias. J Thorac Cardiovasc Surg 1997; 113:836–846.

Ely, JW, Levinson, W, Elder, NC, Mainous, AG III, Vinson, DC. Perceived causes of family physicians' errors. J Fam Pract 1995; 40:337–44.

Enderlen, E, Hotz, G. Beiträge zur Anatomie der Struma und zur Kropfoperation. Z Angew Anat 1918; 3:57–79.

Enker, WE, Merchant, N, Cohen, AM. et al. Safety and efficacy of low anterior resection for rectal cancer: 681 consecutive cases from a specialty service. Ann Surg 1999; 230:544–54.

Epstein, RM, Peters, E. Beyond information. Exploring patient's preferences. JAMA 2009; 302: 195–197.

Esposito, C. Influence of different trocar tips on abdominal wall penetration during laparoscopy. Surg Endosc. 1998; 12:1434.

Fahrtmann, EH, Schoffel, U. Principles and limitations of operative management of intraabdominal infections. World J Surg 1990; 14:210–217.

FAQs. What is Six Sigma? Motorola University, Motorola Inc Web site. http://www.motorola.com/content.jsp?globalObjectId=3088. Accessed on June 14, 2006.

Farke, S, Gögler, H. Anastomoseninsuffizienz nach kontinenzerhaltenden Rektumresektionen. Coloproctology 2006; 22: no 5.

Feldkamp, J, Seppel, T, Becker, A. et al. Jodide or L-thyroxine to prevent recurrent goiter in an iodine-deficient area: prospective sonographic study. World J Surg 1997; 21:10.

Feldman, EA. HIV and blood in Japan: transforming private conflict into public scandal. In: Feldman, EA, Bayer, R. eds. Blood Feuds: AIDS, Blood, and the Politics of Medical Disaster. New York, NY: Oxford University Press; 1999:59–93.

Feldman, EA. Suing doctors in Japan: structure, culture, and the rise of malpractice litigation. In: McCann, M, Engel, D. eds. Fault Lines: Tort Law as Cultural Practice. Stanford, CA: Stanford University (forthcoming, 2009).

Felix, EL, Michas, CA, Gonzalez, MH. Laparoscopic hernioplasty; TAPP vs TEP. Surg Endosc 1995; 9:984.

Felix, EL, Michas, CA, McKnight, RK. Laparoscopic herniorrhaphy; transabdominal preperitoneal floor repair. Surg Endosc 1994; 8:100.

Felix, EL, Scott, S, Crafton, B, Geis, P. et al. Causes of recurrence after laparoscopic hernioplasty. A multicenter study. Surg Endosc 1998; 12:226.

Fellmer, PT, Fellmer, J, Jonas, S. Arzthaftung bei Gallengangsverletzungen nach laparoskopischer Cholezystektomie. Chirurg 2011; 82:68–73.

Femur operation on the wrong side [in Swedish]. Lakartidningen. 1976; 73:1327.

Ferri, EL, Law, S, Wong, KH. et al. The influence of technical complications on postoperative outcome and survival after esophagectomy. Annals of Surgical Oncology 2006; 13/4:557–564.

Ferriman, A. Laparoscopic surgery: two thirds of injuries initially missed. BMJ 2000; 321(7264):784.

Fevang, BT, Fevang, J, Lie, SA. et al. Long-term prognosis after operation for adhesive small bowel obstruction. Ann Surg. 2004; 240:193–201.

Fingerhut, A, Millar, B, Borrie, F. Laparoscopic versus open appendectomy: time to decide: World J Surg 1999; 23:835–845.

Fink, S, Chadhuri, TK. Risk management in suspective acute appendicitis. Perspectives in healthcare risk management 1991; 11:11–4.

Fischer, G, Fetters, MD, Munro, AP, Goldman, E.B. Adverse events in primary care identified from a risk-management database. J Fam Pract 1997; 45:40–6.

Fischer, JE. Is damage to the common bile duct during laparoscopic cholecystectomy an inherent risk of the operation? Am J Surg 2009; 197:829–832.

Fitz, RH. Perforation inflammation of the vermiform appendix with special reference to its early diagnosis and treatment. Am J Med Sci 1886; 92:321–346.

Fitzgibbons, RJ, Jr, Camps, J, Cornet, DA. et al. Laparoscopic inguinal herniorrhaphy. Results of a multicenter trial. Ann Surg 1995, January; 221(1):3–13.

Flaatten, H. The importance of ICN Culture. In: Chiche, J.-D., Moreno, R., Putensen, C. et al. (ed). Patient safety and Quality of Care in Intensive Care Medicine, Berlin, 2009; p. 87–91.

Fletscher, DR, Hobbs, MS, Tan, P. et al. Complications of cholecystectomy: risks of the laparoscopic approach and protective effects of operative cholangiography: a population-based study. Ann Surg. 1999; 229:449–457.

Flowers, L, Riley, T. State-based mandatory reporting of medical errors. An analysis of the legal and policy issues. Portland, ME, National Academy for State Health Policy, 2001.

Flum, DR, Cheadle, A, Prela, C, Dellinger, EP, Chan, L. Bile duct injury during cholecystectomy and survival in medicare beneficiaries. JAMA 2003; 290:2168–2173.

Fowler, DL, White, SA. Laparoscopic-assisted sigmoid resection. Surg Laparosc Endosc 1991; 1:183–8.

Francoeur, JR, Wiseman, K, Buczkowski, AK. et al. Surgeons' anonymous response after bile duct injury during cholecystectomy. Am J Surg 2003; 185:468–475.

Frangou, C. Mayo study counts surgical objects left behind. General Surgery News 2008; 35: 18–19.

Franklin, ME, Rosenthal, D, Abrego-Medina. et al. Prospective comparison of open vs laparoscopic colon surgery for carcinoma. Five-year results. Dis Colon Rectum 1996; 39:10 [Suppl]:35–46.

Fränneby, U, Sandblom, G, Nordin, P. et al. Risk factors for long-term pain after hernia surgery. Ann Surg. 2006; 244:212–219.

Freidson, E. Profession of Medicine: A Study in the sociology of applied knowledge. NY: Harper and Row, 1970; New York.

Freitag, M, Ludwig, K. et al. Klinische und bildgebende Aspekte des Gallensteinileus. Chirurg 1998; 69:265–269.

Frizelle, FA, Hanna, GB. Pelvic abscess following laparoscopic appendectomy [letter]. Surg Endosc 1996; 10:947–948.

Frosch, DL, Kaplan, RM. Shared decision making in clinical medicine: Past research and future directions. Am J Prev Med. 1999; 17:285–294. [PubMed]

Full Disclosure Working Group, Harvard University. When things go wrong: responding to adverse events. March 2006. Available at: www.macoalition.org/documents/respondingToAdverseEvents .pfd. Accessed August 14, 2008.

Furey, A, Stone, C, Martin, R. Preoperative signing of the incision site in orthopaedic surgery in Canada: J Bone Joint Surg Am. 2002; 84-A:1066–1068.

Fusco, MA, Paluzzi, MW. Abdominal wall recurrence after laparoscopic assisted colectomy for de-novo carcinom of the colon. Report of a case. Dis Colon Rektum 1993; 36:858–861.

Gagner, M., Inabnet, B. W. III, Biertho, L. Endoscopic thyroidectomy for solitary nodules. Ann Chir 2003; 128:696–701.

Gallagher, TH, Studdert, D, Levinson, W. Disclosing harmful medical errors to patients. N Engl J Med 2007; 356:2713–2719. Joint Commission on the Accreditation of Healthcare Organization. Hospital Accreditation Standards. Standard RI.2.90 OAK Brook, IL: Joint Commission Resources; 2005.

Gallagher, TH, Waterman, AD, Ebers, AG, Fraser, VJ, Levinson, W. Patient's and physicians' attitudes regarding the disclosure of medical errors. JAMA. 2003; 289:1001–1007. [PubMed].

Gallagher, TH, Waterman, AD, Garbutt, JM, Kapp, JM, Chan, DK, Dunagan, WC, Fraser, VJ, Levinson. W. US and Canadian physicians' attitudes and experience regarding disclosing errors to patients. Arch Intern Med. 2006; 166:1605–1611. [PubMed].

Gandhi, TK, Sittig, DF, Franklin, M, Sussman, AJ, Fairchild, DG, Bates, DW. Communication breakdown in the outpatient referral process. J Gen Intern Med 2000; 15:626–31.

Gardiner, KR, Russell, CF. Thyroidectomy for large multinodular colloid goitre. J R Coll Surg Edinbg. 1995; 40:367–370.

Gawande, AA, Studdert, DM, Orav, EJ, Brennan, TA. et al. Risk factors for retained instruments and sponges after surgery. N Engl J Med 2003; 348:229–235. Comment in: N Engl J Med 2003; 348:1724–5.

Geerdsen, JP, Hee, P. Non toxic goitre. A study of the pituitary thyroid axis in 14 recurrent cases. Acta Chir Scand 1982; 148:221.

Gencosmanoglu, R, Inceoglu, R. An unusual cause of small bowel obstruction: gossypiboma – case report. BMC Surg 2003; 3:6.

Gerber, S, Hämmerli, PA, Glättli, A. Laparoskopische transabdominale präperitoneale Hernioplastik- Evaluation der zugangsbedingten Komplikationen. Chirurg 2000; 71:824.

Germer, CT, Ritz, JP, Buhr, HJ. Laparoskopische Kolonchirurgie. Chirurg 2003; 74:966–982.

Gigerenzer, G Gut feelings: The Intelligence of the Unconscious. New York 2007; Viking Press.

Gigerenzer, G, Brighton, H. Homo heuristicus: why biased minds make better inferences. Top Cogn Sci 2009; 1:107–143.

Gigerenzer, G, Gray, JAM. Better Doctors, Better Patients, Better Decisions. Envisioning Health Care 2020. The MIT Press, Cambridge, Massachusetts, London, England 2011; p 26–27.

Gigot, JF, Etienne, J, Aerts, R, Wibin, E. et al. The dramatic reality of biliary tract injury during laparoscopic cholecystectomy. An anonymous multicenter Begian survey of 65 patients. Surg Endosc 1997; 11:1171.

Gill, BD, Jenkins, JR. Cost-effective evaluation and treatment of the acute abdomen. Surg Clin North Am 1996; 76:71–82.

Giuli, R, Gignoux, M. Treatment of carcinoma of the esophagus. Retrospective study of 2,400 patients. Ann Surg 1980; 192:44–52.

Glassow, F. Short-stay surgery for repair of inguinal hernia. Ann R Coll Surg Engl 1976; 58:133.

Go, PM, Schol, F, Gouma, DJ. Laparoscopic cholecystectomy in the Netherlands. Br J Surg. 1993; 80:1180–1183.

Goldstein, EB. Sensation and perception, 6th ed. Pacific grove, CA: wads worth 2002.

Goligher, JC, Graham, NG, Drukal, FT. Anastomotic dehiscence after anterior resection of rectum and sigmoid. Br J Surg 1970; 57109–19.

Golub, R, Golub, RW, Cantu, R, Stein, HD. A multivariate analysis of factors contributing to leakage of intestinal anastomoses. J Am Coll Surg 1997; 184(4):364–372.

Golub, R, Siddiqui, F, Pohl, D. Laparoscopic versus open appendectomy: a metaanalysis. J Am Coll Surg 1998; 186:545–553.

Gonzalez, AB, Mahesh, M, Kim, KP. et al.: Projected cancer risks from computed tomographic scans performed in the United States in 2007. Arch Intern Med 2009; 169(22):2071–2077.

Gooszen, AW. et al. Operative treatment of acute complications of diverticular disease: primary or secondary anastomosis after sigmoid resection. Eur J Surg 2001; 167:35–39.

Goretzki, PE, Simon, D, Dotzenrath, C. et al. Growth regulation of thyroid and thyroid tumors in humans. World J Surg 2000; 24:193.

Gouzi, JL, Huguier, M, Fagniez, PL. et al. Total versus subtotal gastrectomy for adenocarcinoma of the gastric antrum. A French prospective controlled study. Ann Surg 1989; 209:162–166.

Graff, L, Radford, MJ, Werne, C. Probability of appendicitis before and after observation. Ann Emerg Med 1991; 20:503.

Grant, AM, Scott, NW, O'Dywer, PJ. MRC Laparoscopic Groin Hernia Trial Group. Five-year- follow-up of a randomized trial to assess pain and numbness after laparoscopic or open repair of groin hernia. Br J Surg 2004; 91:1570–1574.

Grant, AM, Scott, NW, O'Dywer, PJ. On behalf of the MRC Laparoscopic Groin Hernia Trial Group Five-year follow-up of a randomized trial to asses pain and numbness after laparoscopic or open repair of groin hernia. Br J of Surg 2004; 91:1570–4.

Greenfield, S, Kaplan, S, Ware, Jr, JE. Expanding patient involvement in care. Effects on patient outcomes. Ann Intern Med. 1985; 102:520–528. [PubMed]

Guller, U, Hervey, S, Purves, H. et al. Laparoscopic versus open appendectomy. Ann Surg 2004; 239:43–51.

Guo, YD, Cai, JF, Chang, YF, Guan, P, Wen, JF. Forensic analysis of 74 tumor related medical mal- practice cases. In: Fa Y., Xue Za Zhi. 2010 Jun; 26(3):192–5.

Gwynn, LK. The Diagnosis of acute appendicitis: clinical assessment versus computed tomography evaluation. J Emerg Med 21:119–123.

Hadrami, J, Rojas, M, de Fenoyl, O. et al. Pulmonary texiloma revealed by haemoptysis 12 years after thoracotomy. Rev Med Interne 1998; 19:826–829.

Hagen, JA, De Meester, SR, Peters, JH, Chandrasoma, P, De Meester, TR. Curative resection for esophageal adenocarcinoma: analysis of 100 en bloc esophagectomies. Ann Surg 2001; 234:520–30.

Hallerback, B, Andersson, C, Englund, N. et al. A prospective randomized study of continuous peritoneal lavage postoperatively in the treatment of purulent peritonitis. Surg Gynecol Obstet 1986; 163:433–436.

Hallfeldt, K, Schmidbauer, S, Trupka, A. Optical trocar types, indications, clinical experiences. Min Invas Ther Allied Technol. 2001; 10:47–50.

Hallfeldt, K, Trupka, A, Kalteis, T. et al. Laparoscopic needles and trocars: an overview of designs and complications. J Laparoendosc. Surg. 1992; 2-117–125.

Hand, AA, Self, ML, Dunn, E. Abdominal wall abscess formation two years after laparoscopic cholecystectomy. Jour Adv Lap Surg 2006; 10:105–107.

Hansis, ML. Begutachtung vorgeworfener Behandlungsfehler – "das gute Gutachten". MED SACH 2006; 102:10–15.

Hardy, KJ. Gallstones and laparoscopic cholecystectomy: a consensus? Aust NZJ Surg. 1994; 64:583–587.

Harrington, JW. Surgical time outs in a combat zone. AORN J. 2009; 89(3):535–537.

Harry, M, Schroeder, R, Hohmann, BJ. Six Sigma: Prozesse optimieren, Null-Fehler-Qualität schaffen, Rendite radikal steigern, 2005. 3rd ed. Frankfurt a.M.

Hartel, W, Dralle, H. Leitlinien zur Therapie der benignen Struma. Grundlagen der Chirurgie – G80. Mitt. Deutsch Ges Chir. 1998; Issue 3.

Hashizume, M, Sugimachi, K. Needle and trocar injury during laparoscopic surgery in Japan. Surg. Endosc. 1997; 11:1198.

Hasson, HM, Rotman, C, Rana, N, Kumari, NA. Open laparoscopy: 29-year-experience. Obstet Gynecol 2000; 96:763–766.

Hau, T, Ohmann, C, Wolmershausen, A. et al. Planned relaparotomy vs relaparotomy on demand in the treatment of intra-abdominal infections. The Peritonitis Study Group of the Surgical Infection Society-Europe. Arch Surg 1995; 130:1193–1196.

Havinghurst, C. Private Reform of tort-law dogma: market opportunities and legal obstacles. Law Contemp. Problems. 1986; 49:143–172.

Haynes, AB, Weiser, TG, Berry, WR. et al. A surgical safety check-list to reduce morbidity and mortality in a global population. N Engl J Med 2009; 360:491–9.

Heald, RJ, Husband, EM, Ryall, RD. The mesorectum in the rectal cancer surgery – the clue to pelvic recurrence? Br J Surg 1982; 69:613–6.

Heald, RJ, Leicester, R. The low stapled anastomoses. Br J Surg 1981; 68:333.

Health and Safety Commission: Third Report: Organizing for Safety, ACSNI, Study Group on Human Factors – HMSO 1993; London.

Heinrich, HW, Granniss, ER. Industrial Accident Prevention, 4th ed. 1959, New York. Cited in: Löber, N. Fehler und Fehlerkultur im Krankenhaus. Gabler Verlag Wiesbaden 2012.

Heise, CP, Starling, JR. Mesh inguinodynia: a new clinical syndrome after inguinal herniorraphy? J Am Surg 1998; 187:514–8.

Hellinger, A, Lange, R, Peitgen, K, Stephan, V. et al. Gallengangsläsionen bei laparoskopischer Cholezystektomie – Rekonstruktionsverfahren und Ergebnisse. Zentralbl Chir 1997; 122:1092.

Helme, S, Samdani, T, Sinha, P. Complications of spilled gallstones following laparoscopic cholecystectomy: a case report and literature overview. J Med Case Reports 2009; 3:8626.

Henne-Bruns, D, Löhnert, M. Aktueller Stand zu Diagnostik und nicht operativen Therapie des Dünndarmileus. Chirurg 2000; 71:503–509.

Henry, JF, Sebag, F. Lateral endoscopic approach for thyroid and parathryoid surgery. Ann Chir 2006; 131:51–56.

Hida, J, Yasutomi, M, Maruyama, T. et al. Lymph node metastases detected in the mesorectum distal to carcinoma of the rectum by the clearing method: justification of total mesorectal excision. J Am Coll Surg 1997; 184:584–8.

Hildebrandt, J, Herrmann, U, Dietrich, H. Der Gallensteinileus und ein Bericht aus 104 Beobachtungen. Chirurg 1990; 61:392.

Hillman, K, Chen, J, Cretikos, M. et al. Introduction of the medical emergency team (MET) System: a cluster-randomized controlled trial. Lancet 2005; 365:2091–2097.

Hip surgery on the wrong-side [in Swedish]. Vardfacket. 1977; 1:68.

Hisham, AN, Azlina, AF, Aina, EN. et al. Total thyroidectomy: the procedure of choice for multinodular goiter. Eur J Surg 2001; 167:403–405.

Hoffmann, J, Jauch, KW. Chirurgie der Appendizitis. In: Bauch, J, Bruch, HP, Heberer, J, Jähne, J (ed). Behandlungsfehler und Haftpflicht in der Viszeralchirurgie. Springer-Verlag 2011; 278–279.

Hofstetter, SR. Acute adhesive obstruction of small intestine. Surg. Gynecol. Obstet. 1981; 152:141.

Hofstetter, W, Swisher, SG, Correa, AM. et al. Treatment outcomes of resected esophageal cancer. Ann Surg 2002; 236:376–84.

Hohenberger, W, Merkel, S. Die laparoskopische Chirurgie des Kolonkarzinoms. Chirurg 2004; 75:1052–1055.

Hohenberger, W. Offene Rektumchirurgie. Chirurg 2007; 78:739–747.

Holden, J, O'Donnell, S, Brindley, J, Miles, L. Analysis of 1263 deaths in four general practices. Br J Gen Pract 1998; 48:1409–12.

Hölscher, U, Laurig, W, Müller-Arnecke, HW. Prinziplösungen zur ergonomischen Gestaltung von Medizingeräten. Bundesanstalt für Arbeitsschutz und Arbeitsmedizin. Berlin, Dresden, 2nd ed. 2008.

Holzheimer, RG, Gathof, B. Re-operation for complicated secondary peritonitis – how to identify patients at risk for persistent sepsis. Eur J Med Res 2003; 8:125–34.

Holzinger, F, Klaiber, C. Trokarhernien. Chirurg 2002; 73:899–904.

Hong, JJ. et al. Prospective study of the incidence and outcome of intra-abdominal hypertension and the abdominal compartment syndrome. Br J Surg 2002; 89:591–596.

Hopkins v., Everad. 80 English Reports 1164 (1615). From: Bal, Sonny, B.: An Introduction to the Medical Malpractice in the United States. In: Clin Orthop Relat Res. 2009; 467 (2): 339–347.

Horwitz, JR, Custer, MD, May, BH, Mehall, JR, Lally, KP. Should laparoscopic appendectomy be avoided for complicated appendicitis in children? J Pediatr Surg 1997; 32:1601–1603.

Hospital Episode Statistics 2005–2006, May, 2009.

Hübler, M, Möllemann, A, Eberlein-Gonska, M. et al. Anonymes Meldesystem kritischer Ereignisse in der Anästhesie – Ergebnisse nach 18 Monaten. Anaesthesist 2006; 55:133–141.

Hübler, M, Möllemann, A, Metzler, H. et al. Fehler und Fehlermeldesysteme in der Anästhesie. Anaesthetist 2007; 56:1067–1072.

Hulscher, JBF, van Sandick, JW, Offerhaus, GJA. et al. Prospective analysis of the diagnostic yield of extended en bloc resection for adenocarcinoma of the esophagus or gastric cardia. Br J Surg 2001; 88:715–719.

Huntington, TR, Klomp, GR. Retained staples as a cause of mechanical small-bowel obstruction. Surg Endosc 1995; 9:353.

Hüttl, TP, Hrdina, C, Geiger, TK, Meyer, G, Schildberg, FW. et al. Management of Common bile duct stones – Results of a nationwide survey with analysis of 8433 common bile duct explorations in Germany. Zentralblatt für Chirurgie 2002; 127:282–288.

Hyodo, M, Hosaya, Y, Hirashima, Y. et al. Minimum leakage rate (0,5%) of stapled esophagojejunostomy with sacrifice of a small part of the jejunum after total gastrectomy in 390 consecutive patients. Dig Surg 2007; 24:269–272.

Hyslop, JW, Maull, KI. Natural history of the retained surgical sponge. South Med J 1982; 75: 657–660.

Ibrahim, JM, Wolodiger, E, Sussman, B. et al. Laparoscopic management of acute small bowel obstruction. Surg. Endosc. 1996; 10:1014–1015.

Ikeda, Y, Takami, H, Sasaki, Y, Takayama, J, Kurihara, H. Are there significant benefits of minimally invasive endoscopic thyroidectomy? World J Surg 2004; 28:1075–1978.

Imhof, M. Behandlungsfehler in der Medizin. Was nun? Schulz-Kirchner-Verlag 2010.

Implementation Planning Study for the Integration of Medical Event Reporting Input and Data Structure for Reporting to AHRQ, CDC, CMS, and FDA. Medstat Report submitted to AHRQ, 2002.

Imran, Y, Azman, MZ. Asymptomatic chronically retained gauze in the pelvic cavity. Med J Malaysia 2005; 60:358–359.

Imren, Y, Rasoglu, I, Ozkose, Z. A different intracardiac mass: retained sponge. Echocardiography 2006; 23:322–323.

Inderbitzi, R, Wagner, HE, Seiler, C. et al. Acute mesenteric ischaemia. Eur J. Surg 1992; 158:123–6.

Ivatury, RR, Nallathambi, M, Rao, PM, Rohman, M, Stahl, WM. Open management of the septic abdomen: therapeutic and prognostic considerations based on APACHE II. Crit Care Med. 1989; 17:511–7.

Jacobs, J, Aland, J, Ballinger, J. Total thyroidectomy: a review of 213 patients. Ann Surg 1983; 197:542.

Jähne, J. Chirurgie der Leistenhernie. Chirurg 2001; 72:456–471.

Jähne, J. Chirurgische Komplikationen. In: Meyer, HJ, Buhr, HJ, Wilke, H (ed). Management des distalen Oesophagus- und Magenkarzinoms. Springer Berlin 2004; p. 325–332.

Jahoda, G. Do we need a Concept of Culture? In: Journal of Cross-Cultural Psychology, 1984, Vol. 15, No 2, p 139–151.

Jamieson, GG, Mathew, G, Lüdemann, R. et al. Postoperative mortality following esophagectomy and problems in reporting its rate. Br Surg 2004; 91:943–947.

Jansen, FW, Kolkman, W, Bakkum, EA. et al. Complications of laparoscopy: an inquiry about closed – versus open – entry technique. Am J Obstet Gynecol 2004; 190:634–638.

Janson, M, Björholt, I, Carlsson, P. et al. Randomized Clinical trial of the costs of open and laparoscopic surgery for colonic cancer. Br J Surg 2004; 91:409–417.

Järvinen, HJ, Luukkonen, P. Sphincter saving surgery for rectal carcinoma. Ann Chir Gynecol 1991; 80:14–8.

Jenkins, DM, Paluzzi, M, Scott, TE. Postlaparoscopic small bowel obstruction. Surg Laparosc Endos 1993; 3:139.

Jensen, JA, Goodson, W. Hopf, HW, Hunt, TK. Cigarette smoking decreases tissue oxygen. Arch Surg 1991; 126:1131.

Jirecek, S, Drager, M, Leitich, H. et al. Direct visual or blind insertion of the primary trocar. Surg Endosc. 2002; 16:626–629.

Johnson, KB, Philips, CA, Orentlicher, D, Hatlie, MJ. A Fault-based administrative alternative for resolving medical malpractice claims. Vanderbilt Law Rev. 1989; 42:1365–1406.

Joint Commission on Accreditation of Healthcare Organizations. Guidelines for implementing the universal protocol for preventing wrong site, wrong procedure, wrong person surgery. JCAHO Web site. http://www.jointcommission.org/PatientSafety/UniversalProtocol/. Accessed June 15, 2006.

Joint Commission on Accreditation of Healthcare Organizations. Sentinel event statistics. December 31, 2005. JCAHO Web site. http://www.jointcommission.org/SentinelEvents/Statistics/. Accessed June 24, 2006.

Joint Commission. Sentinel event statistics. 2007. http://www.jointcommission.org/NR/. Accessed April 24, 2007.

Jonsson, K, Jensen, A, Goodson, WH, Scheuenstuhl, H, West, J, Hopf, HW. Hunt, TK. Tissue oxygenation, anaemia and perfusion in relation to wound healing in surgical patients. Ann Surg 1991; 214:605.

Jorgensen, LN, Kallehave, F, Christensen, E, Siana, JE, Gottrup, F. Less collagen production in smokers. Surgery 1998; 123:450.

Kaiser, CW, Friedman, S, Spurling, KP. et al. The retained surgical sponge: Ann Surg 1996; 224: 79–84. Comment in: Ann Surg 1997; 225:442.

Kaldjian, LC, Jones, EW, Rosenthal, GE, Tripp-Reimer, T, Hillis, SL. An empirically derived taxonomy of factors affecting physicians' willingness to disclose medical errors. J Gen Intern Med. 2006; 21:942–948. [PMC free article] [PubMed].

Kalliomäki, ML, Meyerson, J, Gunnarsson, U. et al. Long-term pain after inguinal hernia repair in a population-based cohort; risk factors and interference with daily activities. Eur J Pain 2008; 12:214–225.

Kang, JY, Ellis, C, Majeed, A. et al. Gallstone – an increasing problem: a study of hospital admissions in England between 1989/1990 and 1999/2000. Aliment Pharmacol Ther. 2003; 17:561–569.

Kant, I, Kritik der praktischen Vernunft, I § 8.

Kapiris, SA, Brough, WA, Royston, CMS, O'Boyle, C, Sedman, PC. Laparoscopic transperitoneal (TAPP) hernia repair – a 7-year two-center experience in 3017 patients. Surg Endosc 2001; 15:972.

Kaplan, HS, Battles, JB, van der Schaaf, TW, Shea, CE, Mercer, SQ. Identification and classification of the causes of events in transfusion medicine. Transfusion 1998; 38:1071–1081.

Karanjia, N, Corder, A, Bearn, P. et al. Leakage from stapled low anastomoses after total mesorectal excision for carcinoma of the rectum. Br J Surg 1994; 81:1224.

Karl, RC, Schreiber, R, Boulware, D, Baker, S, Coppola, D. Factors affecting morbidity, mortality, and survival in patients undergoing Ivor Lewis esophagogastrectomy. Ann Surg 2000; 231:635–643.

Katkhouda, N, Friedländer, MH, Grant, SW, Achanta, KK, Essani, R, Paik, P, Velmahos, G, Campos, G, Mason, R, Mavor, E. Intraabdominal abscess rate after laparoscopic appendectomy. Am J Surg 2000; 180:456–461.

Kato, K, Kawai, T, Suzuki, K. et al. Migration of surgical sponge retained at transvaginal hysterectomy into the bladder: a case report. Hinyokika Klyo 1998; 44(3):183.

Katz, AD, Nemiroff, P. Anastomoses and bifurcations of the recurrent laryngeal nerve – report of 1177 nerves visualized. Am Surg 1993; 59:188–191.

Katz, J. The silent world of doctor and patient. New York: Macmillan, 1982.

Kause, J, Smith, G, Prytherch, D. et al. A comparison of antecedents to cardiac arrest, deaths and emergency intensive care admissions in Australia and New Zealand, and the United Kingdom – the ACADEMIA Study. Resuscitation 2004; 62:275–282.

Kazemier, G, Hof in't, KH, Saad, S. et al. Securing the appendiceal stump in laparoscopic appendectomy: evidence for routine stapling? Surg Endosc 2006; 20:1473–1476.

Keenan, V, Kerr, W, Sherman, W. Psychological Climate and Accidents in an Automotive Plant, In: Journal of Applied Psychology 1951; Vol 35, No 2, p 108–111.

Kern, KA. Malpractice litigation involving laparoscopic cholecystectomy. Cost, cause, and consequences. Arch Surg 1997; 132:392–397. Discussion 397–398.

Kern, KA. Medicolegal analysis of bile duct injury during open cholecystectomy and abdominal surgery. Am J Surg. 1994; 168:217–222.

Kern, KA. Medicolegal analysis of errors in diagnosis and treatment of surgical endocrine disease. Surgery 1993; 114:1167–74.

Kersting, S, Saeger, HD. Akutes Abdomen. In: Bauch, J, Bruch, HP, Heberer, J, Jähne, J. Behandlungsfehler und Haftpflicht in der Viszeralchirurgie. 2011; 323–334.

Kessler, H, Hermanek, Jr. P, Wiebelt, H. Operative mortality in carcinoma of the rectum. Results of the German Multicentre Study. Int J Colorect Dis 1993; 8:158–66.

Keus, F, de Jong, JA, Gooszen, HG, van Laarhoven, CJ. Laparoscopic versus open cholecystectomy for patients with symptomatic cholecystolithiasis. Cochrane Database Syst Rev 2006; CD006231.

Khuri, SF, Daley, J, Henderson, WG. The comparative assessment and improvement of quality of surgical care in the Department of Veterans Affairs. Archives of Surgery, 1998; 228: 491–507.

Khuri, SF, Daley, J, Henderson, WG. The comparative assessment and improvement of quality of surgical care in the Department of Veterans Affairs. Archives of Surgery, 2002; 137:20–27.

Kidney puncture on the wrong-side caution [in Swedish]. Lakartidningen. 1975; 72:793.

Kienzle, HF, Weltrich, H. Lähmung der Stimmbandnerven nach Schilddrüsenresektion. Dtsch Ärztebl. 2001; 98:A43–A46.

Kingham, TP, Pachter, HL. Colonic anastomotic risk factors, diagnosis and treatment. J Am Coll Surg 2009; 208(2):269–278.

Kirstein, H. Der Einfluss Deming auf die Entrichtung des Total Quality Management (TQM), 1994, München.

Kitano, H, Fujimura, M, Kinoshita, T. et al. Endoscopic thyroid resection using cutaneous elevation in lieu of insufflation. Surg Endosc 2002; 16:88–91.

Kitano, S, Iso, Y, Moriyama, M, Sugimachi, K. Laparoscopy-assisted Billroth I gastrectomy. Surg Laparosc Endosc Percutan Tech 1994; 4:146–148.

Kitano, S, Shiraishi, N, Fuji, K. et al. A randomized controlled trial comparing open vs laparoscopy-assisted distal gastrectomy for the treatment of early gastric cancer. An interim report. Surgery 2002; 131 (1 Suppl): 5306.

Kitawaga, Y, Kitano, S, Kubota, T. et al. Minimally invasive surgery for gastric cancer-toward a confluence of two major streams: A review. Gastric Cancer 2005; 8:103–110.

Klaiber, C, Banz, M, Metzger, A. Die Technik der endoskopischen präperitonealen Netzplastik zur Behandlung der Hernien der Leistenregion (TEP). Minim Invasive Chir 1999; 8:86.

Klein, J, Farman, J, Burrell, M. et al. The forgotten surgical foreign body. Gastrointest Radiol 1988; 13(2):173.

Klempa, I. Zeitgemäße Therapie der komplizierten Appendizitis. Chirurg 2002; 73:799–804.

Klinect, JR, Wilhelm, JA, Helmreich, R. Threat and error management: data from line operations safety audits. Proceedings of the 10th International symposium on aviation psychology. Ohio State University, Columbus 1999; pp 683–688.

Klingler, A, Henle, KP, Beller, S, Rechner, J, Zerz, A, Wetscher, GJ, Szinicz, G. Laparoscopic appendectomy does not change the incidence of postoperative infectious complications. Am J Surg 1998; 175:232–235.

Knaus, WA, Draper, EA, Wagner, DP, Zimmermann, JE. APACHE II: a severity of disease classification system. Crit Care Med. 1985; 13:818–829.

Köbberling, J. Das Critical Incident Reporting System (CIRS) als Mittel zur Qualitätsverbesserung in der Medizin. Med Klin 2005; 100:143–148.

Koch, A, Marusch, F, Gastinger, I. Appendizitis: Wann laparoskopisch und wann konventionell operieren? Chir Gastroenterol 2000; 16:126–130.

Kohn, L, Corrigan, JM, Donaldson, MS. To err is human: Building a safer health system. Washington, DC, National Academy Press, 1999.

Kohn, LT, Corrigan, JM, Donaldson, MS (ed). Committee on Quality of Healthcare in America, Institute of Medicine. To Err is Human: Building a safer Health System. Washington DC: National Academy Press; 2000.

Kohn, LT, Corrigan, JM, Donaldson, MS (ed). Committee on Quality in Health Care; Institute of Medicine: to err is human. Building a safer health system. National Academy Press 1999; Washington.

Kohn, LT, Corrigan, JM, Donaldson, MS. To Err is Human: Building a safer Health system. Washington. National Academy Press, 2000.

Kolmorgen, K. Prävention von Laparoskopie-Komplikationen aus gutachterlicher Sicht: Gynäkologie 2002; 35:495–500.

Konishi, I, Watanabe, T, Kishimoto, J, Nagawa, H. Risk factors for anastomotic leakage after surgery for colorectal cancer: results of prospective Surveillance. J Am Coll Surg 2006; 203(3):439–44.

Koperna, T, Schulz, F. Prognosis and treatment of peritonitis. Do we need new scoring systems? Arch Surg 1996; 131:180–186.

Kreis, ME, Jauch, KW. Ileus aus chirurgischer Sicht. Chirurg 2006; 77:883–888.

Kreß, H. Medizinische Ethik. Gesundheitsschutz – Selbstbestimmungsrechte – Heutige Wertkonflikte. 2nd ed. Stuttgart, Kohlhammer, 2009.

Krug, F, Herold, A, Wenk, H, Bruch, HP. Narbenhernien nach laparoskopischen Eingriffen. Chirurg 1995; 66:419.

Kruse, E, Olthoff, A, Schiel, R. Functional anatomy of the recurrent and superior laryngeal nerve. Langenbecks Arch Surg 2006; 391:4–8.

Kukor, JS, Dent, TL. Small intestinal obstruction. In: Nelson, RL, Nyhus, LM. (eds). Surgery of the small intestine. Appleton u. Lange 1987; Norwalk, p 267.

Kwaan, MR, Studdert, DM, Zinner, MJ, Gawande, AA. Incidence, patterns, and prevention of wrong-site surgery. Arch Surg 2006; 141:353–358.

Lacy, AM, Delgado, S, García-Valdecasa, JC. et al. Port-site metasases and recurrence after laparoscopic colectomy. A randomized trial. Surg Endosc 1998 Aug; 12 (8):1039–42.

Lahmann, C, Bergemann, J, Harrison, G, Young, AR. Matrix metalloproteinase-1 and skin ageing in smokers. Lancet 2001; 357:935.

Lai, EC, Lau, WY. Mirizzi syndrome: history, present and future development. ANZ J Surg 2006; 76:251–257.

Lajer, H, Widecrantz, S, Heisterberg, L. Hernias in trocar ports following abdominal laparoscopy. Acta Obstet Gynecol Scand 1997; 76:389.

Lamme, B, Boermaster, MA, Reitsma, JB. et al. Metaanalysis of relaparotomy for secondary peritonitis. Br J Surg 2002; 89:1516–1524.

Lamme, B, Mahler, CW, van Till, JWC. et al. Relaparotomie bei sekundärer Peritonitis. Chirurg 2005; 76:856–867.

Lammers, BJ, Meyer, HJ, Huber, HG. Entwicklungen bei der Leistenhernie vor dem Hintergrund neu eingeführter Eingriffstechniken im Kammerbereich. Nordrhein Chirurg 2001; 72:441–452.

Landercasper, J, Cogbill, TH, Merry, WH. et al. Long-term outcome after hospitalization for small bowel obstruction. Arch Surg. 1993; 128:765–770.

Langwitz, W, Denz, M, Keller, A. et al.: Spontaneous talking time at start of consultation in outpatient clinic. BMJ 2002; 325:682–683.

Lankisch, PG, Mahlke, R, Lübbers, H. Zertifizierte medizinische Fortbildung: Das akute Abdomen aus internistischer Sicht. Dtsch Ärztebl 2006; 103: A-2179/B-1884/C-1821.

Lau, WY, Lai, ECH. Classification of iatrogenic bile duct injury. Hepatobiliary Pancreat Dis Int, Vol 6, N 5, October 15, 2007.

Lauscher, J C, Buhr, HJ, Gröne, J. Erfahrungen aus über 2,100 Hernienreparationen. Chirurg 2011; 82:255–262.

Lauscher, JC, Yafaei, K, Buhr, HJ. et al. Totale extraperitoneale Hernioplastik. Chirurg 2009; 80:956–965.

Lauwers, PR, van Hee, RH. Intraperitoneal gossypibomas: the need of count sponges. World J Surg 2000; 24(5):521.

Law, S, Kwong, DI, Kwok, KF. et al. Improvement in treatment results and long-term survival of patients with esophageal cancer: impact of chemoradiation and change in treatment strategy. Ann Surg 2003; 238:339–47.

Leape, LL. Error in Medicine. JAMA 1994; 272:1851–1857.

Leape, LL. Making health care safe: are we up to it? J Pediatr Surg. 2004; 39:258–268. [PubMed].

Leape, LL. Reporting of adverse events. N Engl J Med 2002; 347(20):1633–1638.

Leape, LL. Reporting of medical errors: time for a reality check. Qual Safety Healthcare. 2000; 9:144–145.

Leape, LL. Why should we report adverse incidents? J Eval Clin Pract. 1999; 5:1–4. [PubMed].

Leflar, RB. Law and patient safety in the United States and Japan. In: Jost, TS (ed). Readings in Comparative Health Law & Bioethics. 2nd ed. Durham, NC. Carolina Academic Press; 2007: 124–126.

Leflar, RB. The Regulation of Medical Malpractice in Japan. Clin Orthop Relat Res. 2009 February; 467 (2):443–449.

Leibl, BJ, Schmedt, CG, Schwarz, J, Kraft, K. et al. Laparoscopic surgery complications associated with trocar tip design: review of literature and own results. J Laparoendosc Adv Surg Tech-Part A, 1999; vol. 9, no. 2, pp.135–140.

Leidel, BA, Kanz, KG. A-B-C-D-E Checkliste verhindert Todesfälle auf Station. In: Notfall Rettungsmed 2010; 13 (8):775–780.

Lembcke, B. Pathophysiologie der gastrointestinalen Ischämie und deren klinische Problematik. Chir Gastroenterologie 2002; 6:529–539.

Leon, EL, Metzger, A, Tsiotos, GG. et al. Laparoscopic management of small bowel obstruction. Indications and outcome. J Gastrointest 1998; Surg 2:132–140.

Leslie, A, Steele, RJ. The interrupted seromucosal anastomoses – still the gold standard. Colorectal Dis 2003; 5:362.

Levy, MM. et al. 2001 SCCM/ESICM/ACCP/ATS/SIS International Sepsis Definitions Conference. Crit Care Med 2003; 31:1250–1256.

Lewis, FR, Holcroft, JW, Boey, J. et al. Appendicitis: a critical review of diagnosis and treatment in 1,000 cases. Arch Surg 1975; 110:677–684.

Liang, M, Lo, K, Marks, JL. Stump appendicitis: a comprehensive review of literature. Am Surg 2006; 72:162–166.

Lichtenstein, EL, Shore, JM. Simplified repair of femoral and recurrent inguinal hernias by a "plug-technic". Am J Surg 1974; 128:439.

Lichtenstein, IL, Shulman, AG, Amid, PK. et al. Cause and prevention of postherniorrhaphy neuralgia: a proposed protocol for treatment. Am J Surg 1988; 155:786–90.

Liem, MS, van der Graaf, Y, van Steensel, CJ. et al. Comparison of conventional anterior surgery and laparoscopic surgery for inguinalhernia repair. N Engl J Med 1997; 336:1541–7.

Lillemoe, KD, Melton, GB, Cameron, JL. et al. Postoperative bile duct strictures: management and outcome in the 1990s. Ann Surg. 2000; 232:430–441.

Lillemoe, KD. To err is human, but should we expect more from a surgeon? Ann Surg 2003; 237:470–471.

Lincourt, AE, Harrell, A, Cristiano, J, Sechris, C. et al. Retained foreign bodies after surgery. Journal of Surgical Research 2007, Volume 138, Issue 2, p. 170–171.

Lippert, H, Koch, A, Marrusch, F, Wolff, S, Gastinger, I. Offene – versus laparoskopische Appendektomie. Chirurg 2002; 73:791–798.

Liu, Q, Djuricin, G, Prinz. RA. Total thyroidectomy for benign thyroid disease. Surgery 1998; 132:2–7.

Livingstone, EH, Rege, RV. Technical Complications are arising as common duct exploration is becoming rare. Journal of the American College of Surgeons, 2005; 201:426–433.

Lo, B. Resolving Ethical Dilemmas: A Guide for Clinicians, 2nd ed. Lippincott: Williams and Wilkins, Philadelphia, 2000.

Löber, N. Fehler und Fehlerkultur im Krankenhaus. Gabler Verlag Wiesbaden 2012.

Lock, G. Akute mesenteriale Ischämie – häufig übersehen und häufig fatal. In: Medizinische Klinik 2002; 97:402–409.

Loos, MJ, Roumen, RM, Scheltinga, MR. Chronic sequelae of common elective groin hernia repair. Hernia 2007; 11:169–173.

Lörken, M, Marnitz, U, Schumpelick, V. Freier intraperitonealer Clip als Ursache eines mechanischen Dünndarmileus. Chirurg 1999; 70:1492–1493.

Luketich, JD, Alvelo-Rivera, M, Buenaventura, PO, Christie, NA, Mc Caughan, JS, Little, VR. et al. Minimally-invasive esophagectomy. Outcomes in 222 patients. Ann Surg 2003; 238:486–494.

Lustosa, SA, Matos, D, Atallah, AN, Casto, AA. Stapled versus handsewn methods for colorectal anastomoses surgery. Cochrane Database Syst Rev. 2001; (3):DC003144.

Madariaga, JR, Dodson, SF, Selby, R, Todo, S. et al. Corrective treatment and anatomic considerations for laparoscopic cholecystectomy injuries. J Am Coll Surg: 1994 September; 179(3): 321–325.

Makary, MA, Mukherjee, A, Sexton, JB. et al. Operating room briefings and wrong-site surgery. J Am Coll Surg 2007; 204(2):236–243.

Makary, MA, Sexton, JB, Freischlag, JA. et al. Patient safety in surgery. Ann Surg 2006; 243(5):628.

Makeham, MA, Dovey, SM, County, M, Kidd, MR. An international taxonomy for errors in general practice: a pilot study. Med J Aus 2002; 177:62–63.

Mäkelä, JT, Kiviniemi, H, Laitinen, S. Risk factors for anastomotic leakage after left-sided colorectal resection with rectal anastomoses. Dis Colon Rectum 2003; 46(5):653–660.

Mangano, DT, Layug, EL, Wallace, A, Tateo, I. Effect of atenolol on mortality and cardiovascular morbidity after noncardiac surgery. Multicenter Study of Perioperative Ischemia. Research Group. N Engl J Med 1996; 335:1713–1720.

Manner, M, Stickel, W. Diagnostik bei Verdacht auf Appendicitis – Lässt sich eine Appendicitis sonographisch ausschließen? Chirurg 2001; 72:1036–1042.

Marcy, PY, Hericord, O, Novellas, S. Lymph node-like lesion of the neck after pharyngolaryngectomy. AJR Am J Roentgenol 2006; 1878:W135–W136.

Margenthaler, JA, Walter, E, Katherines, L. et al. Risk factors for adverse outcomes after the surgical treatment of appendicitis in adults. Ann Surg 2003 July; 238(1):59–66.

Marinker, M, Shaw, J. Not to be taken as directed. BMJ 2003; 326:348–349.

Marshall, JC. et al. Multiple organ dysfunction score: a reliable descriptor of a complex clinical outcome. Crit Care Med 1995; 23:1638–1652.

Martens, MF, Hendriks, T. Postoperative changes in collagen synthesis in intestinal anastomoses of the rat: differences between small and large bowel. Gut 1991; 32(12):1482–1487.

Mason, LB. Migration of surgical sponge into small intestine. JAMA 1968; 205(13):938.

Massaron, S, Bona, S, Fumaqalli U. et al. Long-term sequelae after 1,311 primary inguinal hernia repairs. Hernia 2008; 12:57–63.

Massarweh, N.N, Flum DR. Role of intraoperative cholangiography in avoiding bile duct injury. J Am Coll Surg. 2007; 204:656–664.

Matthiesen, P, Hallböök, O, Rutegard, J. et al. Defunctioning stoma reduces symptomatic anastomotic leakage after low anterior resection of the rectum for cancer: a randomized multicenter trial. Ann Surg 2007; 246(2):207–14.

Maxwell, JM, Ragland, JJ. Appendicitis. Improvements in diagnosis and treatment. Am Surg 1991; 57:282–285.

May, T, Aulisio, MP. Medical malpractice mistake prevention, and compensation. Kennedy Inst. Ethics J. 2001; 11:134–146.

Mazor, KM, Reed, GW, Yood, RA, Fischer, MA, Baril, J, Gurwitz, JW. Disclosure of medical errors: what factors influence how patients respond? J Gen Intern Med 2006; 21(7):704–10.

Mc Burney, C. The incision made in the abdominal wall in cases of appendicitis, with a description of a new method of operating. Ann Surg 1894; 20:38–43.

Mc Cormack, K, Scott, NW, Go, PM, Ross, S. et al. The EU Trialists Collaboration laparoscopic techniques versus open techniques for inguinal hernia repair. Cochrane Database. Syst Rev. 2003: CD001785.

Mc Donald K. et al., Measures of patient safety based on hospital administrative data: the patient safety indicators. Rockville, MD. Agency for Healthcare Research and Quality, 2002.

Mc Lean, TR. Risk management observations from litigation involving laparoscopic cholecystectomy. Arch Surg 2006; 141:643–648.

Mc Wilson, LR, Runciman, WB, Gibberd, RW. et al. The quality in Australian health care study. Med J Aust 1995; 163:458–471.

Meinberg, EG, Stern, PJ. Incidence of wrong-site surgery among hand surgeons. J Bone Joint Surg [Am] 2003; 85:193–197.

Melton, GB, Lillemoe, KD, Cameron, JL. et al. Major bile duct injuries associated with laparoscopic cholecystectomy: effect of surgical repair on the quality of life. Ann Surg 2002; 235:888–895.

Memon, MA. Laparoscopic appendectomy current status. Ann R Coll Surg Eng 1997; 79:393–402.

Menegaux, F, Turpin, G, Dahman, M. et al. Secondary thyroidectomy in patients with prior thyroid surgery for benign disease: a study of 203 cases. Surgery 1999; 125:479–483.

Meyer, HJ, Sauer, P. Postoperative Probleme nach Magenresektion oder Gastrektomie und Pankreasresektion. Gastroenterologe 2009; 4:437–445.

Meyer-Marcotty, W, Plarre, I. Die chronische Appendizitis. Langenbecks Archives of Surgery 1986; 369:187.

Miettinen, P, Pasanen, P, Lahtinen, J, Alhava, E. Acute abdominal pain in adults. Ann Chir Gynaecol 1996; 85:5–9.

Miller, G, Boman, J, Shrier, I. et al. Etiology of small bowel obstruction. Am J Surg 2000; 180:33–36.

Miller, G, Boman, J, Shrier, I. et al. Natural history of patients with adhesive small bowel obstruction. Br J Surg 2000; 87:1240–1247.

Millikan, KW, Silverstein, J, Hart, V. et al. A 15-year review of esophagectomy for carcinoma of the esophagus and cardia. Arch Surg 1995; 130:617–24.

Milsom, JW, Böhm, B, Hammerhofer, KA, Fazio V. et al. A prospective, randomized trial comparing laparoscopic versus conventional techniques in colorectal cancer surgery: a preliminary report. JAMA Coll Surg 1998; 187:55–7.

Minnesota Department of Health. Adverse health events in Minnesota: second annual public report. [Minnesota Department for Health Web site]. February 2006: Available at www.health. state.mn.us/patientsafety/ae/aereport0206.pdf. Accessed April 24, 2007.

Mirkovitch, V, Cobo, F, Robinson, JWL, Menge, H, Combo, SZ. Morphology and function of the dog ileum after mechanical occlusion. Clin Sci Med 1976; 50:123.

Miserez, M, Alexandre, JH, Campanelli, G. et al. The European hernia society groin hernia classification: Simple and easy to remember. Hernia. 2007; 11:113–116.

Mishra, A, Agarwal, A, Agarwal, G, Mishra, SK. Total thyroidectomy for benign thyroid disorders in an endemic region. World J Surg 2001; 25:307–310.

Mishra, R. Wrong girl gets tonsils taken out. Boston Globe. December 23, 2000; Section B:1.

Missbach-Kroll, A, Nussbaumer, P, Kuenz, M. et al. Critical incident reporting system. Chirurg 2005; 76:868–875.

Mittelpunkt, A, Nora, PF. Current features in the treatment of acute appendicitis: an analysis of 1,000 cases. Arch Surg 1966; 60:971–975.

Möllemann, A, Eberlein-Gonska, M, Koch, T, Hübler, M. Klinisches Risikomanagement – Implementierung eines anonymen Fehlermeldesystems in der Anästhesie eines Universitätsklinikums. Anaesthesist 2005; 54:377–384.

Montz, FJ, Holschneider, CH, Munro, MG. Incisional hernia following laparoscopy: a survey of the American association of gynaecologic laparoscopists. Obstet Gynecol 1994; 84:881.

Mouhsine, E, Halkic, N, Garofalo, R. et al. Soft-tissue textiloma: a potential diagnostic pitfall. Can J Surg 2005; 48:495–496.

Mouret, P. How I developed laparoscopic cholecystectomy. Ann Acad Med Singapore 1996; 25:744–747.

Mucha, Jr. P. Small intestinal obstruction. Surg Clin North Am 1987; 67:597–620.

Mughal, MM, Bancewicz, J, Irving, MH. Laparostomy: a technique for the management of intractable intra-abdominal sepsis. Br J Surg 1986; 73:253–259.

Mühe, E. [Laparoscopic cholecystectomy – late results]. Klin Chir. 1991: 10–13.

Mühe, E. [Laparoscopic cholecystectomy – late results]. Langenbecks Arch Chir Suppl Kongressbd. 1991:416–423.

Mühe, E. Long-term follows-up after laparoscopic cholecystectomy. Endoscopy 1992; 24:754–758.

Mulier, S, Penninckx, F, Verwaest, C, Filez, L, Aerts, R, Fieuws, S. et al. Factors affecting mortality in generalized postoperative peritonitis: multivariate analysis in 96 patients. World J Surg. 2003; 27:379–84.

Murthy, SC, Law, S, Whooley, BP. et al. A trial fibrillation after esophagectomy is a marker for postoperative morbidity and mortality. J Thorac Cardiovasc Surg 2003; 126(4):1162–1167.

Mussack, T, Trupka, AW, Schmidbauer, S, Hallfeldt, KKJ. Zeitgerechtes Management von Gallengangkomplikationen nach laparoskopischer Cholezystektomie. Chirurg 2000; 71: 174–181.

Nakeeb, A, Comuzzie, AG, Martin, L. et al. Gallstones. Genetics versus environment. Ann Surg. 2002; 235:842–849.

National Coordinating Council for Medication Error Reporting and Prevention, USA. NCC MERP Taxonomy of Medication Errors. 1998. http://www.nccmerp.org/taxo0731.pdf. Accessed 3 June 2003.

National Patient Safety Agency National Reporting and Learning System. Dataset (http://npsa.nhs.uk/dataset/dataset.asp.accessed) on 9 November 2005.

National Practitioner Data Bank Public Data file: Available online at: www.npdb-hipdb.hrsa.gov/pubs/stats/Public_Use_Data:_File.pdf. Last accessed on July 28, 2008.

Nelson, H, Sargent, DJ, Wieland, S. et al. A comparison of laparoscopically assisted and open colectomy for colon cancer. N Engl J Med 2004; 350:2050–2059.

Neu, J. Ärztliche Sorgfalt, Fahrlässigkeit, Behandlungsfehler, In: Neu, J., Petersen, D., Schellmann, WD (ed). Arzthaftung, Arztfehler, Darmstadt 2001; p. 429–431.

Neuhaus, P, Schmidt, SC, Hintze, RE, Adler, A, Veltzke, W, Raakow, R. et al. Classification and treatment of bile duct injuries after laparoscopic cholecystectomy. Chirurg 2000; 71:166–173.

Nguyen, DB, Silen, W, Hodin, RA. Appendectomy in the pre- and postlaparoscopic eras. J Gastrointest Surg 1999; 3:67–73.

NIH Consensus Conference. Gallstones and laparoscopic cholecystectomy. JAMA 1993; 269:1018–1024.

NJW 2000; p. 1749.

Nyhus, LM, Condon, RE. Hernia 4th ed. Lippincott Philadelphia 1995.

O'Dowd, TC. Five years of heartsink patients in general practice. BMJ 1988 Aug 20–27; 297:528–30.

O'Leary, DS, Jacott, WE. Mark my limb. AHRQ Morbidity & Mortality Rounds on the Web. December 2004. http://webmm.ahrq.gov/case.aspx?caseID=82. Accessed August 28, 2005.

Ockert, D, Bergert, H, Knopke, R, Saeger, HD. Das akute Abdomen. Gynäkologe 2003; 35:336–339.

Ohgami, M, Otani, Y, Kumai, K. et al. Curative laparoscopic surgery for early gastric cancer. Five years experience. World J Surg 1999; 23:187–192.

OLG Hamm. Ruling of the Higher District Court (OLG) Hamm from 28.11.2008, file reference 26 and 28/08. In: GesR 2009:247–248.

OLG Schleswig-Holstein. Ruling of the Higher District Court (OLG) Schleswig-Holstein from 29.5.2009, file reference 4 V 38108.

Orlando, R, Palatini, P, Lirussi, F. Needle and trocar injuries in diagnostic laparoscopy under local anaesthesia: what is the true incidence of these complications? Laparoendosc Adv Surg Tech 2003; A 13:181.

Orlando, R, 3rd, Russel, JC, Lynch, J. et al. Laparoscopic cholecystectomy: a state-wide experience: the Connecticut Laparoscopic Cholecystectomy Registry. Arch Surg. 1993; 128:494–498.

Orringer, MB, Marshall, B, Iannettoni, MD. Transhiatal esophagectomy: clinical experience and refinements. Ann Surg 1999; 230:392–400.

Ortega, AE, Hunter, JG, Peters, JH, Swanstrom, LL, Schirmer, BA. Prospective, randomised comparison of laparaoscopic appendectomy with open appendectomy. Am J Surg 1995; 169:208–212.

Oussoultzoglu, E, Panaro, F, Rosso, E. et al. Use of BiClamp decreased the severity of hypocalcemia after total thyroidectomy compared with LigaSure: a prospective study. World J Surg 2008; 32:1968–1973.

Pacelli, F, Doglietto, GB, Alfieri, S, Piccioni, E, Sgadari, A, Gui, D. et al. Prognosis in intra-abdominal infections. Multivariate analysis on 604 patients. Arch Surg 1996; 131:641–5.

Paes, E, Vollmar, J.F, Hutschenreiter, S, Schoenberg, M.H, Schölzel, E. Diagnostik und Therapie des akuten Mesenterialinfarkts. Chir. Gastroenterologie 1990; 6:473–480.

Page, B, Paterson, C, Young, D, O'Dywer, PJ. Pain from primary inguinal hernia and the effect of repair on pain. Br J Surg 2002; 89:1315–1318.

Paik, PS, Towson, JA, Anthone, GJ, Ortega, AE, Simons, AJ, Beart, RW. Intraabdominal abscesses following laparoscopic and open appendectomies. J Gastrointest Surg 1997; 1:188–192.

Pakkastie, T, Luukkonen, P, Järvinen, HJ. Anastomotic leakage after anterior resection of the rectum. Eur J Surg 1994; 160:293.

Palanivelu, C, Prakash, A, Senthilkumar, R, Senthilnathan, P, Parthasarathi, R, Rajan, S. et al. Minimally invasive esophagectomy: thorascopic mobilization of the esophagus and mediastinal lymphadenectomy in prone position – experience of 130 patients. J Am Coll Surg 2006; 203:7–16.

Palazzo, FF, Sebag, F, Henry, JF. Endocrine surgical technique, endoscopic thyroidectomy via the lateral approach. Surg Endosc 2006; 20:339–342.

Pande, PS, Neumann, RP, Cavanagh, RR. The Six Sigma way: How GE, Motorola and other top companies are honing their performance. McGraw-Hill Professional, 2000; New York.

Pankaj, GR, Soonawalla, ZF, Grant, HW. Medico legal costs of bile duct injuries incurred during laparoscopic cholecystectomy. HPB (Oxford). 2009; March; 11 (2):130–134.

Panzica, M, Krettek, C, Cartes, M. "Clinical Incident Reporting System" als Instrument des Risikomanagements für mehr Patientensicherheit. Unfallchirurg 2011; 114:758–767.

Pappalardo, G, Guadalaxara, A, Frattaroli, FM. et al. Total compared which subtotal thyroidectomy in benign nodular disease: personal series and review of published reports. Eur J Surg 1998; 164:501.

Park, K. Human error. In: Salvendy G (ed). Handbook of human factors and ergonomics. Willey, New York, 1997; pp 150–173.

Park, YL, Han, WK, Bae, WG. 100 cases of endoscopic thyroidectomy: breast approach. Surg Laparosc Endosc Percutan Tech 2003; 13:20–25.

Patankar, SK, Larach, SW, Ferrara, A. et al. Prospective comparison of laparoscopic vs. open resections for colorectal adenocarcinoma over a ten-year period. Dis Colon Rectum 2003; 46(5):601–611.

Patient Safety and Quality Improvement Act, 119, Stat 424, 2005. In: Kalra, De Gruyter, p. 88.

Patient safety first alert – implementing a correct site surgery policy and procedure. AORN J 2002; 76:785–788.

Pellegrini, CA, Thomas, MJ, Way, LW. Recurrent biliary stricture. Patterns of recurrence and outcome of surgical therapy. Am J Surg 1983; 147:175.

Perissat, J, Collet, D, Belliard, R. Gallstones. Laparoscopic treatment – cholecystectomy, cholecystostomy, and lithotripsy. Our own technique. Surg Endosc. 1990; 4:1–5.

Perrow, C. Normal accidents. Living with high-risk technologies. Princeton, N.J., Princeton University Press, 1999.

Perzik, SL, Katz, B. The place of total thyroidectomy in the management of thyroid disease. Surgery 1967; 62:436.

Physician Insurers Association of America. Rockville, M.D.: Physician Insurers Association of America Laparoscopic Procedure Study.

Pichlmayr, R, Lehr, I, Pahlow, J, Guthy, E. Postoperative continuous open dorsoventral abdominal lavage in severe forms of peritonitis. Chirurg 1983; 54:299–305.

Pidgeon, N. Safety Culture: Key Theoretical Issues. In: Work and Stress, 1998; Vol 12, No 3, p 202–216.

Pieper, R, Kager, L, Nasman, P. Acute appendicitis: a clinical study of 1,018 cases of emergency appendectomy. Acta Chir Scand 1982; 148:51–62.

Pittman-Waller, VA, Myers, JG, Stewart, RM. et al. Appendicitis: why so complicated? Analysis of 5,755 consecutive appendectomies. Am Surg 2000; 66:548–443.

Plaus, WJ. Laparoscopic trocar site hernias. J Laparoendosc Surg 1993; 3:567.

Polat, A, Nayci, A, Polat, G, Aksoyek, S. Dexamethasone down-regulated endothelial expression of intercellular adhesion molecule and impairs healing of bowel anastomoses. Eur J Surg 2002; 168:500.

Polk, HC. Quality, safety and transparency. Ann Surg 2005; 242:293–301. [PMC free article] [PubMed]

Poobalan, AS, Bruce, J, King, PM. et al. Chronic pain and quality of life following open inguinal hernia repair. Br J Surg 2001; 88:1122–1126.

Post, S, Schuster, KL. Verlassenes, Bewährtes und Aktuelles zu operativer Dünndarmileus-Therapie. Chirurg 2000; 71:524–531.

President's Commission for the Study of Ethical Problems in Medicine and Biomedical Research. The ethical and legal implications of informed consent in the patient-practitioner relationship. Volume one: report: Washington, DC: U.S. Government Printing Office, 1982.

Putzki, H, Reichert, B. Does measuring of axillorectal temperature difference help in the diagnosis of acute appendicitis? Langenbecks Arch Chir 1988; 373:310–312.

Radbruch, G. Die peinliche Gerichtsordnung Kaiser Karl V. von 1532 (Carolina). Stuttgart: Reclam-Universal-Bibliothek, 1967.

Radiation given to wrong patient. The Gazette. December 2, 1992; Section A:3.

Rall, M, Dieckmann, P., Stricker, E. Arbeitsgruppe Incident Reporting innerhalb des Forums Qualitätssicherung und Ökonomie des BDA und der DGAI. Patientensicherheits-Optimierungs-System (PaSOS) – Das neue bundesweite Incident-Reporting-System von DGAI/BDA. Anaesth Intensivmed 2006; 47:520–524.

Rall, M, Gaba, DM. Human performance and patient safety. In: Miller, RD (ed) Miller's anesthesia. Elsevier Churchill Livingston, Philadelphia, 2005; p. 3021–3071.

Rall, M, Martin, J, Geldner, G. et al. Charakteristika effektiver Incident-Reporting-Systeme zur Erhöhung der Patientensicherheit. Anaesthesiol Intensivmed 2006; 47:9–19.

Rall, M. et al. Patient safety and errors in medicine: development, prevention and analyses of incidents. Anaesthesiol Intensivmed Notfallmed Schmerzther 2001; 36(6):321–330.

RAND Cooperation for the European Commissions: Technical report: Improving patient safety in the EU, 2008. URL: www.Rand.Org.com.

Ranking tables for states: population in 2000 and population change from 1990 to 2000 (PHC-T-2). US Census Bureau Web site. Revised July 31, 2002. http://www.census.gov/population/www/cen2000/phc-t2.html. Accessed June 16, 2006.

Rappaport, W, Haynes, K. The retained surgical sponge following intra-abdominal surgery. A continuing problem. Arch Surg 1990; 125(3):405.

Rasmussen, J, Duncan, K, Leplat, J. New Technology and Human Error, Chichester 1986.

Rasmussen, J. Human Errors. A Taxonomy for Describing Human Malfunction in industrial installations, In: Journal of Occupational Accidents, 1982; Vol. 4, No.2–4, p. 311–333.

Rastogi, V, Dy, V. Simple technique for proper approximation and closure of peritoneal and rectus sheat defects at port site after laparoscopic surgery. J Laparoendosc Adv Surg Techn 2001; A 11:13.

Raute, M, Podlech, P, Jaschke, W, Manegold, BC. et al. Management of bile duct injury and strictures following cholecystectomy. World J Surg 1993; 17:553.

Reason, JT. Human Error. Cambridge; Cambridge University Press.

Reason, JT. Human error: models and management. BMJ 2000; 320:768–770.

Reason, JT. Managing the Risks of Organizational Accidents, Aldershot 1997.

Reason, JT. Menschliches Versagen: Psychologische Risikofaktoren und moderne Technologien, Heidelberg 1994.

Reason, JT. Understanding Adverse Events: Human factors. In: Quality and Safety in Health Care, 1995; Vol 4, no 2, p. 80–89.

Rees, AM. Communication in the physician-patient relationship. Bull Med. Libr Assoc, 1993 January; 81(1).

Reeve, TS, Delbridge, L, Lohen, A. et al. Total thyroidectomy: the preferred option for multinodular goiter. Ann Surg 1987; 206:782–786.

Reid, RI, Dobbs, BR, Frizelle, FA. Risk factors for post-appendectomy intra-abdominal abscess. Aust NZ J Surg 1999; 69; 373–374.

Reiertsen, O, Trondsen, E, Bakka, A, Andersen, OK, Larsen, S, Rosseland, AR. Prospective non-randomized study of conventional versus laparoscopic appendectomy. World J Surg 1994; 18:411–416.

Renzulli, P, Krähenbühl, L, Sadowski, C, Al-Adili, F. et al. Moderne diagnostische Strategie beim Ileus. Zentralbl Chir 1998; 123:1334.

Repair of groin hernia with synthetic mesh: Meta-analysis of randomized controlled trials. Ann Surg 2002; 235:322–332.

Reuter, F. Vermeidung von Eingriffsverwechslungen. Unfallchirurg 2009, 112:675–678.

Revesz, G, Siddiqi, TS, Buchheit, WA, Bonitatibus, M. Detection of retained surgical sponges. Radiology 1983; 149(2):411.

Rexer, M, Ditterich, D. Rupprecht, H. Vakuumtherapie bei kolorektaler Anastomoseninsuffizienz. Coloproctology 2004; 26:285–290.

Ribalta, T, McCutcheon, IE, Neto, AG. et al. Textiloma (gossypiboma) mimicking recurrent intracranial tumor. Arch Pathol Lab Med 2004; 128:749–758.

Ridings, P, Evans, DS. The transabdominal pre-peritoneal (TAPP) inquinal hernia repair: a trip along the learning curve. IR Coll Surg Edingb 2000; 45:29.

Rioux, M. Sonographic detection of the normal and abnormal appendix. Am J Roentgenol 1992; 158:773.

Risher, WH, McKinnon, WM. Foreign body in the gastrointestinal tract: intraluminal migration of laparotomy sponge. South Med J 1991; 84(8):1042.

Ritz, JP, Runkel, N, Berger, G. et al. Prognosefaktoren des Mesenterialinfarktes. Zentralbl. Chir. 1997; 122:332–8.

Robbennolt, JK. Apologies and Medical Error. Clin Orthop Relat Res. 2009 February; 467(2): 376–382.

Robbennolt, JK. Apologies and settlement levers. J Empir Legal Studies. 2006; 3:333–373.

Röher, HD, Horster, FA, Frilling, A. et al. Morphologie und funktionsgerechte Chirurgie verschiedener Hyperthyreoseformen. Chirurg 1991; 62:176.

Roscher, R, Frank, R, Baumann, A, Beger, HG. Chirurgische Behandlungsergebnisse beim mechanischen Dünndarmileus. Chirurg 1991; 62:614.

Roslyn, JJ, Binns, GS, Hughes, EF. et al. Open cholecystectomy: a contemporary analysis of 42,474 patients. Ann Surg. 1993; 218:129–137.

Roumen, RM, Weerdenburg, HP. MR features of a 24-year-old gossypiboma. A case report. Acta Radiol 1998; 39:176–178.

Roy, PG, Soonawalla, ZF, Grant, H. Medico legal costs of bile duct injuries incurred during laparoscopic cholecystectomy. HPB (Oxford), 2009 March; 11(2):130–134.

Ruling of the Higher District Court (OLG) Hamm from 28.11.2008, file reference 26 and 28/08. In: GesR 2009:247–248.

Ruling of the Higher District Court (OLG) Schleswig-Holstein from 29.05.2009, file reference 4 V 38108. In: OLG Schleswig 2009:594–597.

Runciman, WB, Helps, SC, Sexton, EJ. et al. A classification for incidents and accidents in the healthcare system. J Qual Clin Pract 1998; 18:199–211.

Runciman, WB. Lessons from the Australian Patient Safety Foundation: setting up a national patient safety surveillance system – is this the right model? Quality and Safety in Health Care, 2002; 11:246–251.

Rusnak, RA, Borer, JM. et al. Misdiagnosis of acute appendicitis: common features discovered in cases after litigation. Am J Emergency Med 1994; 12:397–403.

Russell, JC, Walsh, SJ, Mattie, AS, Lynch, JT. Bile duct injuries, 1989–1993. A state-wide experience. Connecticut laparoscopic cholecystectomy registry. Arch Surg. 1996; 131:382–388.

Rutkow, JM. Epidemiologic, economic and sociologic aspects of hernia surgery in the United States in the 1990s. Surg Clin North Am 1998; 78:941–951.

Rybowiak, V, Garst, H, Frese, M. et al. Error Orientation Questionnaire (EOQ): Reliability, Validity, and Different Language Equivalence, In: Journal of Organizational Behaviour 1999; Vol 20, no 4, p 527–547.

Sakari, H. Report on the Nationwide Incidence of Medical Accidents: III [in Japanese]. Tokyo, Japan: Japan Ministry of Health, Labour & Welfare; 2006; 18.

Salzgeber, F. Kunden- und Prozessorientierung in Versicherungsunternehmen, Karlsruhe 1996; 209–228.

Sarda, AK, Pandey, N, Neogi, S, Dhir, U. Postoperative complications due to a retained surgical sponge. Singapore Med J 2007; 48(6):e160.

Sasako, M, Sano, T, Yamamoto, S. et al. Left thoracoabdominal approach versus abdominal-transhiatal approach for gastric. Cancer of the cardia or subcardia: A randomized controlled trial. Lancet Oncol 2006; 7:644–651.

Sauer, M, Jarrett, JC. Small bowel obstruction following diagnostic laparoscopy. Fertil Steril 1984; 42:653.

Sauerland, S, Lefering, R, Neugebauer, EA. Laparoscopic versus open surgery for suspected appendicitis (Cochrane Review) [In Process Citation]. Cochrane Database Syst Rev 2002; CD001546.

Schäfer, M, Lauper, M, Krähenbühl, L. Trocar and Veress needle injuries during laparoscopy. Surg Endosc 2001; 15:275.

Schaller, G, Kuenkel, M, Manegold, BC. Serious trocar accidents in laparoscopic surgery: a French survey of 103,852 operations. Surg Laparosc Endosc 1996; 6:367.

Schein, M, Wittmann, DH, Aprahamian, CC. et al. The abdominal compartment syndrome: the physiological and clinical consequences of elevated intra-abdominal pressure. J Am Surg 1995; 180:745–753.

Schein, M. Management of severe intra-abdominal infection. Surg Annu 1992; 24 Pt 1:47–68.

Schein, M. Planned reoperations and open management in critical intra-abdominal infections: prospective experience in 52 cases. World J Surg 1991; 15:537–545.

Schein, M. Schein's Common sense emergency abdominal surgery. Springer, Berlin, Heidelberg, New York, 2000.

Schick, KS, Hüttl, TP, Fertmann, JM. et al. A critical analysis of laparoscopic appendectomy: how experience with 1,400 appendectomies allowed innovative treatment to become standard in a university hospital. World J Surg 2008; 32:1406–1413.

Schiedeck, THK. et al. Laparoscopic surgery for the cure of colorectal cancer. Dis Colon Rectum 2000; 431–438.

Schimmel, EM. The hazards of hospitalisation. Ann Intern Med 1964; 60:100-110. In: Cohen, D. Maßnahmen zur Verbesserung der Patientensicherheit. Bundesgesundheitsbl 2011; 54:171–175.

Schmedt, CG, Leibl, BJ, Däubler, P, Bittner, R. Access-related complications – analysis of 6,023 consecutive laparoscopic hernia repairs. Min invas. The Allied Technol 2001; 10:23–30.

Schmidt, SC, Langrehr, JM, Hintze, RE, Neuhaus, P. Long term results and risk factors influencing outcome of major bile duct injuries following cholecystectomy. Br J Surg 2005; 93:76–82.

Schneider, PM, Müller, MK, Schiesser, M. Chirurgische Therapiestrategien beim Oesophagus-Magenkarzinom. Gastroenterologe 2009; 4:209–223.

Schneller, ES, Wilson, NA. Professionalism in 21th century Professional Practice: Autonomy and Accountability in Orthopaedic Surgery. Clin Orthop Relat Res 2009 October; 467(10):2561–2569.

Schönleben, K, Strobel, A, Schönleben, F, Hoffmann, A. Belassene Fremdkörper aus der Sicht des Chirurgen. Chirurg 2007; 78:712.

Schröder, FH, Hugosson, J, Roobol, MJ. et al.: Screening and prostate-cancer mortality in a randomized European Study. N Engl J Med 2009; 360(13):1320–1328.

Schulte, KM, Röher, HD. Behandlungsfehler bei Operationen an der Schilddrüse. Chirurg 1999; 70:1131–1138.

Schultz, C, Baca, I, Götzen, V. Laparoscopic inguinal hernia repair – a review of 2,500 cases. Surg Endosc 2001; 15:582.

Schultz, RJ, Whitfield, GF, LaMura, JJ. et al. The role of physiologic monitoring in patients with fractures of the hip. J Trauma 1985; 25:309–316.

Schumpelick, V, Töns, C, Kupcyk-Joeris, D. Operation der Leistenhernie, Klassifikation, Verfahren-swahl, Technik und Ergebnisse. Chirurg 1991; 62:641.

Schumpelick, V. Leistenbruchreparation nach Shouldice 1984; Chirurg 55:25–28.

Schüttelkopf, E. Erfolgsstrategie Fehlerkultur. In: Ebner, G, Heimerl, P, Schüttelkopf, EM (ed). Fehler-Lernen-Unternehmen: Wie Sie die Fehlerkultur und Lernreife Ihrer Organisation wahrnehmen und gestalten. Frankfurt a.M. 2008; p. 151–314.

Schwappach, DL, Koeck, CM. What makes an error unacceptable? A factorial survey on the disclosure of medical errors. Int J Qual Health Care. 2004; 16(4):317–26. [PubMed]

Schwender, T. Organisationsfehler aus der Sicht des Chefarztes. Gynäkologe 1999; 32:927–932.

Schwerk, WB. Ultrasound first in acute appendix? Unnecessary laparotomies can often be avoided. Muench Med Wschr 2000; 142:29–32.

Scott, NW, McCormack, K, Graham, P. Open mesh versus non-mesh for repair of femoral and inguinal hernia. Chochrane Database Syst Rev 2002; CD002197.

Scurr, JRH, Brigstocke, JR, Shields, DA. et al. Medico legal claims following laparoscopic cholecystectomy in the UK and Ireland. Ann R Coll Surg Engl. 2010; 92:286–291.

Sebag, F, Palazzo, FF, Harding, J. et al. Endoscopic lateral approach thyroid obectomy: safe evolution from endoscopic parathyroidectomy. World Surg 2006; 30:802–805.

Seedhouse, D. Liberating medicine. Chichester: Wiley, 1991; 119.

Seiden, SC, Barach, P. Wrong-side/wrong-site, wrong-procedure, and wrong-patient adverse events. Archives of Surgery, 2006; vol 141, No 9:931–939.

Seligman, K. License revoked for embryo mix-up. San Francisco Chronicle. March 31, 2005; B.4. http://sfgate.com/cgi-bin/article.cgi?file=/c/a/2005/03/31/BAGIOC10PK1.DTL. Accessed November 28, 2005.

Semm, K. Endoscopic appendectomy. Endoscopy 1983; 15:59–64.

Senagore, A, Milsom, JW, Walshaw, RK, Dunstan, R, Mazier, WP, Chaudry, IC. Intramural pH: a quantitative measurement for predicting colorectal anastomotic healing. Dis Colon Rectum 1990; 33:175.

Shields, R. The absorption and secretion of fluid and electrolytes in the obstructed bowel. Br J Surg 1965; 52:774.

Shojania, KG, Duncan, BW, McDonald, KM. et al. eds. Making Healthcare Safer: A Critical Analysis of Patient Safety Practices. Subchapter 43.2. Strategies to avoid wrong-site surgery. Evidence Report/Technology Assessment No. 43, AHRQ Publication No. 01-E058. Rockville. MD: Agency for Healthcare Research and Quality; 2001; 498–503.

Sicklich, JK, Camps, MS, Lillemoe, KD, Melton, GB. et al. Surgical management of bile duct injuries sustained during laparoscopic cholecystectomy. Ann Surg. 2005; Vol 241, No 5.

Siewert, JR, Hölscher, AH, Becker, K. et al. Cardia Cancer: Attempt at a therapeutically relevant classification. Chirurg 1987; 58:25–32.

Siewert, JR, Stein, HJ, Bartels, H. Insuffizienzen nach Anastomosen im Bereich des oberen Gastrointestinaltrakts. Chirurg 2004; 75:1063–1070.

Siewert, JR. Oesophaguskarzinom. Onkologe 2007; 13:949–960.

Sigman, HH, Fried, GM, Garzon, J. et al. Risks of blind versus open approach to celiotomy for laparoscopic surgery. Surg Laparos Endosc 1993; 3:296.

Silberman, VA. Appendectomy in a large metropolitan hospital. Retrospective analysis of 1,013 cases. Am J Surg 1981; 142:616–618.

Silen, W. Strangulation obstruction of the small intestine. Arch. Surg. 1962; 85:137.

Sivovich, B, Welch, H. Cervical cancer screening among women without a cervix. JAMA 2004; 291:2990–2993.

Slotema, ETh, Sebag, F, Henry, JF. What is the Evidence for Endoscopic Thyroidectomy in the Management of Benign Thyroid Disease? Word J Surg 2008; 32(7):1325–1332.

Smith, C. Surgical tools left in five patients. Available online at: http://seattlepi.nwsource.com/local/49883_error08.shtml. Last accessed on March 12, 2008.

Smith, GB, Prytherch, DR. et al. A review, a performance evaluation, of single-parameter "track and trigger" Systems. Resuscitation 2008; 79:11–21.

Soop, M, Fryksmark, U, Köster, M, Haglund, B. The incidence of adverse events in Swedish hospitals: a retrospective medical record review study. Int J Qual Health Care 2009; 21:285–291.

Sorensen, LT, Jorgensen, T, Kirkeby, LT, Skovdal, J, Vennits, B, Wille-Jorgensen, P. Smoking and alcohol abuse are major risk factors for anastomotic leakage in colorectal surgery. Br J Surg 1999; 86:927.

Sosa, JA, Bowman, HM, Tielsch, JM. et al. The importance of surgeon experience for clinical and economic outcomes from thyroidectomy. Ann Surg 1998; 228:320–330.

Spom, E, Petroski, GF, Mancini, GJ. et al. Laparoscopic appendectomy – Is it worth the cost? Trend analysis in the US from 2000 to 2005. J Am Coll Surg 2009; 208:179–185.

Stahel, PhF, Sabel, AL, Victoroff, MS. et al. Wrong-site and wrong-patient procedures in the Universal Protocol Era. Arch Surg 2010; 145(10):978–984.

Stawicki, SP, Cipolla, J, Bria, C. Comparison of open abdomens in non-trauma and trauma patients: a retrospective study: OPUS 12 Scientist 2007; 1(1):1–8.

Stawicki, SP, Evans, DC, Cipolla, J. et al. Retained surgical foreign bodies: A comprehensive review of risks and preventive studies. Scandinavian Journal of Surgery 2009; 98:8–17.

Steel, K, Gertman, PM, Crescenzi, C. et al. Iatrogenic illness on a general medical service at a university hospital. N Engl J Med 1981; 304:638–642.

Steinmüller, T, Ulrich, R, Rayes, N. et al. Operationsverfahren und Risikofaktoren in der Therapie der benignen Struma multinodosa. Chirurg 2001; 72:1453.

Stevenson, FA, Barry, CA, Britten, N, Barber, N, Bradley, CP. Doctor-patient communication about drugs: the evidence for shared decision making. Soc Sci Med. 2000; 50:829–840. [PubMed]

Stewart, L, Robinson, TN, Lee, CM, Liu, K, Whang, K, Way, LW. Right hepatic artery injury associated with laparoscopic bile duct injury: incidence, mechanism, and consequences. J Gastrointest Surg 2004; 8:523–531.

Stewart, RM, Corneille, MG, Johnston, JJ. et al.: Transparent and open Discussion of Errors does not increase Malpractice Risk in Trauma Patients. Ann Surg 2006 May; 243(5):645–651.

Stoppa, RE, Rives, JL, Warlaumont, CR. et al. The use of Dacron in the repair of hernias of the groin surgery. Clin North Am 1984; 64:269.

Stoppa, RE, Warlaumont, CR. The peritoneal approach and prosthetic repair of the groin hernia. In: Nyhus, LM, Condon, RE. (eds) Hernia, 3rd ed. Lippincott, Philadelphia 1989; p 199.

Storfer, M.D. Problems in left-right discrimination in a high-IQ population. Perception Mot Skills. 1995; 81:491–497.

Strasberg, SM, Brunt, LM. Rationale and use of the critical view of safety in laparoscopic cholecystectomy. J Am Coll Surg 2010; 211:132–138.

Strasberg, SM, Hertl, M, Soper, NJ. An analysis of the problem of biliary injury during laparoscopic cholecystectomy. J Am Coll Surg. 1995; 180:101–125.

Strasberg, SM. Biliary injury in laparoscopic surgery: part 1. Processes used in determination of standard of care in misidentification injuries. J Am Coll Surg. 2005; 201:598–603.

Strasberg, SM. Biliary injury in laparoscopic surgery: part 2. Changing the culture of cholecystectomy. J Am Coll Surg. 2005; 201:604–611.

Strasberg, SM. Error traps and vasculo-biliary injury in laparoscopic and open cholecystectomy. J Hepatobiliary Pancreat Surg 2008; 15:284–292.

Strelec, SR. Anaesthesia and surgery: not always a one-sided affair. ASA Newsletter. http://www.asahg.org/Newsletters/1996/06_96/feature4htm. Accessed November 28, 2005.

Stricker, E, Rall, M, Siegert, N. et al. Das Patienten-Sicherheits-Informations-System PaSIS. Ein internet-basiertes interaktives Meldesystem für negative und positive Ereignisse in der Anästhesie. Intensiv- und Notfallmedizin. In: Jäckel, A (ed). Telemedizinführer. Medizin-Forum 2006; Ober-Mörlen, p. 67–77.

String, A, Berber, E, Foroutani, A. et al. Use of the optical access trocar for safe and rapid entry in various laparoscopic procedures. Surg Endosc. 2001; 15:570–573.

Strobel, C, Büchler, MW. Chirurgische Therapie der Peritonitis. Chirurg 2011; 82:242–248.

Studdert, DM, Mello, MM, Brennan, TA. Medical malpractice. N Engl J Med 2004; 350:283–290. [PubMed]

Studdert, DM, Mello, MM, Gawande, AA, Brennan, TA, Wang, YC. Disclosure of medical injury to patients: an improbable risk management strategy. Health Aff (Millwood). 2007; 26(1):215–26. [PubMed]

Stumpf, M, Klinge, U, Mertens, PR. Prognostische Faktoren. Chirurg 2004; 75:1056–1062.

Sturm, J, Post, S. Benigne Erkrankungen der Gallenblase und Gallenwege. Chirurg 2000; 71: 1530–1551.

Sykes, PA, Boulter, KH, Schofield, PF. Small bowel microflora in acute intestinal obstruction and Crohn's disease. Br J Surg 1974; 52:774.

Tacyildiz, I, Aldemir, M. The mistakes of surgeons: "gossypiboma". Acta Chir Belg 2004; 104: 71–75.

Takami, HE, Ikeda, Y. Minimally invasive thyroidectomy. Curr Opin Oncol 2006; 18:43–47.

Takami, HE, Ikeda, Y. Total endoscopic thyroidectomy. Asian J Surg 2003; 26:82–85.

Tan, GH, Gharib, H. Thyroid incidentalomas: management approaches to non-palpable nodules discovered incidentally on thyroid imaging. Ann Intern Med 1997; 126:226–231.

Tang, E, Ortega, AE, Anthone, GJ, Beart, RWJ. Intraabdominal abscesses following laparoscopic and open appendectomies. Surg Endosc 1996; 10:327–328.

Tate, JJT, Chung, SCS, Dawson, J, Leong, HT, Chan, A, Lau, WY, Li, AKC. Conventional versus laparoscopic surgery for acute appendicitis. Br. J Surg 1993; 80:761–764.

Teichmann, W, Wittmann, DH, Andreone, PA. Scheduled reoperations (etappenlavage) for diffuse peritonitis. Arch Surg 1986; 121:147–152.

Teixeira, PG, Inaba, K, Salim, A. et al. Retained foreign bodies after emergent trauma surgery: incidence after 2526 cavitary explorations. Am Surg 2007; 73:1031–1034.

Telem, DA, Chin, EH, Nguyen, SQ. Risk factors for anastomotic leak following colorectal surgery. Arch Surg 2010; 145(4):371–376.

The Hammurabi Code and the Sinaitic Legislation. Chilperic, E (ed). London, 1921.

Thomas, P, Doddoli, C, Lienne, P. et al. Changing patterns and surgical results in adenocarcinoma of the oesophagus. Br J Surg 1997; 84:119–25.

Thompson, HJ, Jones, PF. Active observation in adults with abdominal pain. Am J Surg 1986; 152:522.

Thomusch, Q, Sekulla, C, Dralle, H. Rolle der totalen Thyreoidektomie im primären Therapiekonzept der benignen Knotenstruma. Chirurg 2003; 74:437–442.

Toellner, R. Illustrierte Geschichte der Medizin. Vol. I, Andreas u. Andreas Verlagsbuchhandlung Salzburg, 1986.

Tonouchi, H, Mohri, Y, Tanaka, K. et al. Diagnostic sensitivity of contrast swallow for leakage after gastric resection. World J Surg 2006; 31:128–131.

Tsiotos, GG, Luque-de Leon, E, Soreide, JA, Bannon, MP, Zietlow, SP, Baerga-Varela, Y. et al. Management of necrotizing pancreatitis by repeated operative necrosectomy using a zipper technique. Am J Surg 1998; 175:91–8.

Ulsenheimer, K. Belassene Fremdkörper aus der Sicht des Juristen. Chirurg 2007; 78:28–34.

Ulsenheimer, K. Der Behandlungsfehler aus juristischer Sicht: Zivilrechtlicher Schadensersatz – gerichtliche Strafverfahren, In: Wolff, H (ed). Der chirurgische Behandlungsfehler. Teupitzer Gespräche 2001; Heidelberg 2002; p. 3.

University of California at San Francisco-Stanford University. Evidence-based Practice Center. Making Health Care Safer: A Critical Analysis of Patient Safety Practices. Report No. AHRQ 01-E508. Rockville, MD: Agency for Healthcare Research and Quality, 2001.

Ureter surgery of the wrong side [in Swedish]. Tidskr Sver Sjukskot. 1975; 42:62.

Vader, VL, Vogt, DM, Zucker, KA, Thilstead, JP, Curet, MJ. Adhesion formation in laparoscopic inguinal hernia repair. Surg Endosc 1997; 11:825.

Valente, JF, Hricik, D, Weigel, K. et al. Comparison of sirolimus vs. mycophenolate mofetil on surgical complications and wound healing in adult kidney transplantation. Am J Transplant 2003; 3:1128.

van Geloven, AW, Biesheuvel, TH, Luitse, JSK, Hoitsma, HFW, Obertop, H. Hospital admissions of patients aged over 80 years with acute abdominal complaints. Eur J Surg 2000; 166: 866–871.

van Sandick, JW, van Lanschot, JJ, ten Kate, FJ, Tijssen, JG, Obertop, H. Indicators of prognosis after transhiatal esophageal resection without thoracotomy for cancer. J Am Coll Surg 2002; 194(1):28–36.

van Veen, RN, Wijsmuller, AR, Vrijland, WW. et al. Randomized clinical trial of mesh versus non-mesh primary inguinal hernia repair: Long-term chronic pain at 10 years. Surgery 2007; 142: 695–698.

van Westreenen, M. et al. Influence of peroperative lavage solutions on peritoneal defence mechanisms in vitro. Eur J Surg 1999; 165:1066–1071.

Velanovic, V, Morton, JM, McDonald, M. Analysis of the SAGES outcomes initiative cholecystectomy, registry. Surg Endosc 2006; 20:43–50.

Vignali, A, Fazio, VW, Lavery, IC. et al. Factors associated with the occurrence of leaks in stapled rectal anastomoses: a review of 1,014 patients. J Am Coll Surg 1997; 185(2):105–113.

Vincent, C, Neale, G, Woloshynowych, M. Adverse events in British hospitals: preliminary retrospective record review, BMJ 2001; 322:517–519.

Vincent, JL. et al. The SOFA (Sepsis-related Organ Failure Assessment) score to describe organ dysfunction/failure. On behalf of the Working Group of Sepsis-Related Problems of the European Society of Intensive Care Medicine. Intensive Care Med. 1996; 22:707–710.

Vinz, H. Communication from the Conciliation Body of the Northern German State Chamber of Medicine. Schleswig-Holsteinisches Ärzteblatt 2002; 06.

von Rahden, BHA, Stein, HJ, Siewert, JR. Barrett's Esophagus and Barrett's Cancer. Curr Oncol Rep 2003; 5:203–209.

Vries de, EN, Ramrattan, MA, Smorenburg, SM. et al. The incidence and nature of in-hospital adverse events: a systematic review. Qual Safe Health Care. 2008 June, 17 (3):216–223.

Wacha, H, Hau, T, Dittmer, R, Ohmann, C. Risk factors associated with intraabdominal infections: a prospective multicenter study. Peritonitis Study Group. Langenbecks Arch Surg 1999; 384:24–32.

Wachter, RM. Focus Patientensicherheit. ABW Wissenschaftsverlag 2008.

Wadman, M, Syk, I, Elmstahl, S. Survival after operations for ischaemic bowel disease. Eur J Surg 2000; 166:872–877.

Walsh, DC, Roediger, WE. Stump appendicitis – a potential problem after laparoscopic appendectomy. Surg Laparoscop Endosc 1997; 7:357–358.

Walsh, RM, Henderson, JM, Vogt, DP, Mayes, JT, Grundfest-Broniatowski, S. et al. Trends in bile duct injuries from laparoscopic cholecystectomy. J Gastrointest Surg. 1998; 2:458–462.

Walter, P, Lindemann, W, Koch, B, Feifel, G. Der akute Mesenterialinfarkt. Klinikarzt 1992; 21:4457–463.

Wassenaar, EB, Raymakers, JT, Rakia, S. Fatal intestinal ischemia after laparoscopic correction of incisional hernia. JSLS 2007; Jul-Sept; 11(3):389–393.

Way, S, Stewart, L, Gantert, W. et al. Causes and prevention of laparoscopic bile duct in juries: analysis of 252 cases from a human factors and cognitive psychology perspective. Ann Surg 2003; 237:460–469.

Weeks, JC, Nelson, H, Gelber, S. et al. Short-term quality-of-life-outcomes following laparoscopic assisted colectomy vs open colectomy for colon cancer. A randomized trial. JAMA 2002; 287:321–328.

Weeks, WB, Foster, T, Wallace, AE. et al. Tort Claims Analysis in the Veteran Health Administration for Quality Improvement. The Journal of Law. Medicine & Ethics 2001; 29:335–345.

Weingart, SN, Wilson, RM, Gibberd, RW, Harrison, B. Epidemiology of medical error. BMJ 2000; 320:730.

Weiser, ThG, Haynes, AB, Lashoher, A. et al. Perspectives in quality: designing the WHO Surgical Safety checklist. International Journal for Quality in Health Care. 2010; Vol 22, No 5.

Weithorn, LA, Scherer, DG. Children's involvement in research participation decisions: psychological considerations. In: Grodin, MA, Glantz, LH. eds. Children as Research Subjects. New York, NY: Oxford Press. 1994; 133–180.

Welsch, T, von Frankenberg, M, Büchler, MW. et al. Diagnostik und Definition der Nahtinsuffizienz aus chirurgischer Sicht. Chirurg 2001; 82:48–55.

Weltrich, H. Offenbarungspflicht bei ärztlichen Behandlungsfehlern? Gynäkologe 2004; 37: 277–278.

Wexner, SD, Cohen, SM. Port site metastases after laparoscopic colorectal surgery for cure of malignancy. Br J Surg 1995; 82:295–8.

Wheeler, MH. Total thyroidectomy for benign thyroid disease. Lancet 1998; 35:1626–1627.

Wherry, DC, Marohn, MR, Malanoski, MP. et al. An external audit of laparoscopic cholecystectomy in the steady state performed in medical treatment facilities of the Department of Defense. Ann Surg. 1996; 224:145–154.

Wherry, DC, Rob, CG, Marohn, MR. et al. An external audit of laparoscopic cholecystectomy performed in medical treatment facilities of the Department of Defense. Ann Surg. 1994; 220: 626–634.

White, GE. Tort law in America: An Intellectual History. New York, NY: Oxford, V. Press; 2003.

Wichmann, MW, Meyer, G, Angele, MK. et al. Recent advances in minimally invasive colorectal cancer surgery. Onkologe 2002; 25:318–323.

Wienke, A, Janke, K. Darstellung des Nervus recurrens bei einer Schilddrüsenoperation. Widerstreit zwischen chirurgischer Schule und HNO-Schule. Urteil des OLG Düsseldorf vom 25.01.2007 – I-8 U 115/05. Laryngo-Rhino-Otol 2007; 80:595–596.

Wig, JD, Goenka, MK, Suri, S. et al. Retained surgical sponge: an unusual cause of intestinal obstruction. J Clin Gastroenterol 1991; 24(1):57.

Wilde, J. PSA screening cuts deaths by 20%, says world's largest prostate cancer study. ERSPC Press Office 2009; Carver Wilde Communications.

Willis, S, Stumpf, M. Insuffizienzen nach Eingriffen am unteren Gastrointestinaltrakt. Chirurg 2000; 75:1071–1078.

Witman, AB, Park, DM, Hardin, SB. How do patients want physicians to handle mistakes? A survey of internal medicine patients in an academic setting. Arch Intern Med. 1996; 156(22): 2565–9.

Wolf, AM, Henne-Bruns, D. Anastomoseninsuffizienz im Gastrointestinaltrakt. Chirurg 2002; 73:394–407.

Woods, MS, Traverso, LW, Kozarek, RA. et al. Biliary tract complications of laparoscopic cholecystectomy are detected more frequently with routine intraoperative cholangiography. Surg Endosc. 1995; 110:1076–1080.

World alliance for patient safety. WHO draft guidelines for adverse event reporting and learning system – from information to action. http://www.who.int/patientsafety/events/05/Reporting-Guidelines.pdf.

World Health Organization: WHO draft guidelines for adverse event reporting and learning systems. 2005; WHO/EIP/SPO/QPS/05.3, Geneva.

Wright, D, Paterson, C, Scott, N, Hair, A, O'Dywer, PJ. Five-Year Follow-Up of Patients Undergoing Laparoscopic or Open Groin Hernia Repair. A Randomized Controlled Trial. Ann of Surg 2002; 235:333–7.

Wright, O. Wrong embryos implanted in three patients. The Times (London). October 29, 2002; Home news: 4.

Wu, AW, Cavanaugh, TA, McPhee, SJ, Lo, B, Micco, GP. To tell the truth: ethical and practical issues in disclosing medical mistakes to patients. J Gen Intern Med 1997; 12(12):770–5. [PMC free article]

Wu, AW, Huang, JCh, Stokes, S. et al. Disclosing Medical Errors to Patients: It's not what you say, it's what they hear. J Gen Int Med. 2009 September; 24(9):1012–1017.

Wu, AW. Medical error: the second victim. The doctor who makes the mistakes needs help too. BMJ 2000; 320:726.

Xiaohang, L, Jialin, Z, Lixuan, S. et al. Laparoscopic versus conventional appendectomy – a meta-analysis of randomized controlled trials. BMC Gastroenterol 2010; 10:129.

Xie, ZG, Zheng, J. Autopsy study of 275 medical dispute cases. Zhonghua Bing Li Xue Za Zhi. 2009 Jun; 38 (6):370–5.

Yalçin, B, Ozan, H. Relationship between the Zuckerkandl's tubercle and entrance point of the inferior laryngeal nerve. Clin Anat 2007; 20:640–643.

Yalçin, B, Poyrazoglu, Y, Ozan, H. Relationship between the Zuckerkandl's tubercle and the inferior laryngeal nerve including the laryngeal branches. Surg Today 2007; 37:109–113.

Yalçin, B, Tunali, S, Ozan, H. Extralaryngeal division of the recurrent laryngeal nerve: a new description for the inferior laryngeal nerve. Surg Radiol Anat 2008; 30:215–220.

Yildirim, S, Tarim, A, Nursal, TZ. et al. Retained surgical sponge (gossypiboma) after intraabdominal or retroperitoneal surgery: 14 cases treated at a single centre. Langenbecks Arch Surg 2006; 391(4):390.

Zambudio, AR, Rodriquez, JR, Riquelme, J. et al. Prospective Study of postoperative Complications after total thyroidectomy for multinodular goiters by surgeons with experience in Endocrine Surgery. Ann Surg 2004 July; 240(1):18–25.

Zegers, M, de Bruijne, MC, Wagner, C. et al. Adverse events and potentially preventable deaths in Dutch hospitals: results of a retrospective patient record review study. Qual Saf Health Care 2009; 18:297–302.

Zhang, H, Wiegmann, DG, Thaden, TL. et al. Safety Culture: A Concept in Chaos? In: Human Factors and Ergonomics Society (ed). Proceedings of the 46th Annual Human Factors and Ergonomics Society Meeting, Santa Monica 2002; p 1404–1408.

Zielke, A. Appendizitis. Chirurg 2002; 73:782–790.

Index